Radiology at a Glance

Radiology at a Glance

Rajat Chowdhury

MA (Oxon), MSc, BM BCh, MRCS
Specialist Registrar in Clinical Radiology
Southampton General Hospital, UK
Chair of the British Institute of Radiology Trainee Committee

Iain D. C. Wilson

MEng (Oxon), BMedSci, BM BS, MRCS
Specialist Registrar in Clinical Radiology
Southampton General Hospital, UK

Christopher J. Rofe

BSc, MB BCh, MRCP
Specialist Registrar in Clinical Radiology
Southampton General Hospital, UK

Graham Lloyd-Jones

BA, MB BS, PCME, MRCP, FRCR
Consultant Radiologist
Salisbury District Hospital, UK

WILEY-BLACKWELL

A John Wiley & Sons, Ltd., Publication

This edition first published 2010, © 2010 by Rajat Chowdhury, Iain Wilson, Christopher Rofe, Graham Lloyd-Jones

Blackwell Publishing was acquired by John Wiley & Sons in February 2007. Blackwell's publishing program has been merged with Wiley's global Scientific, Technical and Medical business to form Wiley-Blackwell.

Registered office: John Wiley & Sons Ltd, The Atrium, Southern Gate, Chichester, West Sussex, PO19 8SQ, UK

Editorial offices: 9600 Garsington Road, Oxford, OX4 2DQ, UK
                       The Atrium, Southern Gate, Chichester, West Sussex, PO19 8SQ, UK
                       111 River Street, Hoboken, NJ 07030-5774, USA

For details of our global editorial offices, for customer services and for information about how to apply for permission to reuse the copyright material in this book please see our website at www.wiley.com/wiley-blackwell

Library of Congress Cataloging-in-Publication Data

Radiology at a glance / Rajat Chowdhury . . . [et al.].
    p. ; cm. – (At a glance series)
  Includes index.
  ISBN 978-1-4051-9220-0
1. Radiology, Medical–Outlines, syllabi, etc.   I. Chowdhury, Rajat.   II. Series: At a glance series (Oxford, England)
  [DNLM: 1. Diagnostic Imaging. WN 180 R12885 2010]
  R896.5.R33 2010
  616.07′54–dc22

                                                               2009035145

ISBN: 9781405192200

A catalogue record for this book is available from the British Library.

Set in 9 on 11.5 pt Times by Toppan Best-set Premedia Limited
Printed and bound in Singapore by Fabulous Printers Pte Ltd

1   2010

Contents

Foreword

As a medical student in the early 1970s I rarely ventured to the X-ray department, which seemed a dark and mysterious place. However, change was in the air. CT and ultrasound were beginning to make their mark and were revolutionising the management of patients. More and more often, erudite discussions on the ward ended with 'let's see what the radiologists think'.

Imaging is rapidly replacing the physician's palpating hand and the needle is taking the place of the surgeon's scalpel. The transition is not yet complete but the trend is clear: diagnostic imaging and interventional radiology are playing an increasingly important role in diagnosis and therapy and are set to determine the flow of patients through 21st century hospitals. It is, therefore, essential that medical students and young doctors become more familiar with the opportunities that modern imaging can offer.

This excellent book by Drs Rajat Chowdhury, Iain Wilson, Christopher Rofe and Graham Lloyd-Jones manages to cover all the essential aspects of modern imaging. Its approach is particularly suited to the intended readership, as the emphasis is on the most important findings and on the impact of radiology on clinical practice rather than on radiological minutiae. *Radiology at a Glance* is an excellent guide on how best to use a radiology department, and to request the diagnostic imaging test that is likely to provide the answer to the clinical condition being investigated. It also covers essential aspects of radiological technology, to help demystify modern imaging techniques, and provides a very necessary understanding of radiation protection. The increasingly important role of interventional radiology is also explained, as well as the opportunities it offers to replace traditional surgical techniques for many conditions.

I am sure that this book will be a very valuable companion to traditional medical textbooks and that it will help medical students and young doctors become more effective in their work by using modern radiology departments to the best advantage of their patients.

Andy Adam
President of The Royal College of Radiologists
Professor of Interventional Radiology, Guy's King's and
St. Thomas' School of Medicine, University of London

Preface and Acknowledgements

The *at a Glance* series has served us well through our careers and we felt that it was time that the specialty of radiology was also given the *at a Glance* treatment. We present *Radiology at a Glance* in this classic style to help teach the basics of radiology in a simple and clear fashion. Since the GMC published 'Tomorrow's Doctors' in 1993, medical schools have restructured their curricula to include clinically integrated teaching. This has meant detailed factual learning has been replaced with a more focused and clinically orientated medical course, including radiological images from the outset of the programme. With this in mind, we have also included radiological anatomy and covered conditions that regularly appear in medical school exams. These 'classic cases' are found in separate chapters allowing easy access for doctors on the wards.

We have written this book not only with medical students and junior doctors in mind, but trust that it will be a useful aid to students of radiography, nursing and physiotherapy, as well as other health professionals. We therefore hope it will be a valuable tool in gaining an understanding of the essentials of clinical radiology.

We would like to express our gratitude to all the consultants and teachers at Southampton General Hospital and to the Wessex Radiology Training Programme for their inspiration, meticulous teaching and expert guidance. We extend warm thanks to Professor Andy Adam for giving his precious seal of approval for this venture. We would also like to thank our publishers, in particular Ben Townsend and Laura Murphy, for showing such enthusiasm for all our ideas and turning them into reality. We would like to dedicate this book to our families who have supported us through this great experience. Finally, we thank all our readers for taking the time to read this book, and in return we hope you feel it was time well spent.

Rajat Chowdhury
Iain D. C. Wilson
Christopher J. Rofe
Graham Lloyd-Jones

Abbreviations

#	fracture
AAA	abdominal aortic aneurysm
ACL	anterior cruciate ligament
ADC	apparent diffusion coefficient
ALARA	as low as reasonably achievable
AP	anterior to posterior
APTT	activated partial thromboplastin time
ARDS	acute respiratory distress syndrome
ARSAC	Administration of Radioactive Substances Advisory Committee
ATLS	Advanced Trauma Life Support
AVN	avascular necrosis
AXR	abdominal X-ray
Ba	barium
CIN	contrast-induced nephropathy
CBD	common bile duct
COPD	chronic obstructive pulmonary disease
CPPD	calcium pyrophosphate dehydrate
CR	computed radiography
CSF	cerebrospinal fluid
CT	computed tomography
CTA	computed tomographic angiography
CTKUB	computed tomography of kidneys, ureters and bladder
CTPA	computed tomographic pulmonary angiography
CXR	chest X-ray
DEXA	dual energy X-ray absorptiometry
DIC	disseminated intravascular coagulation
DIPJ	distal interphalangeal joint
DMSA	dimercaptosuccinic acid
DOB	date of birth
DP	dorsal to plantar
DR	digital radiography
DRUJ	distal radioulnar joint
DTPA	diethylene triamine pentaacetic acid
DVT	deep vein thrombosis
DWI	diffusion-weighted (magnetic resonance) imaging
Echo	echocardiography
EDH	extradural haemorrhage/haematoma
eGFR	estimated glomerular filtration rate
EndoUS	endoultrasound
ERCP	endoscopic retrograde cholangiopancreatography
EVAR	endovascular aneurysm repair
FB	foreign body
FDG	fluorodeoxyglucose
FEV_1	forced expiratory volume in 1st second
FLAIR	fluid attenuated inversion recovery
FVC	forced vital capacity
FNAC	fine-needle aspiration cytology
GI	gastrointestinal
GORD	gastro-oesophageal reflux disease
HIV	human immunodeficiency virus
HRCT	high resolution computed tomography
IBD	inflammatory bowel disease
ICD	implantable cardioverter defibrillator
ICH	intracerebral haemorrhage
ICP	intracranial pressure
ID	identification details
INR	international normalised ratio
IR	interventional radiology
IR(ME)R 2000	Ionising Radiation (Medical Exposure) Regulations 2000
IRR99	Ionising Radiation Regulations 1999
IV	intravenous
IVC	inferior vena cava
IVU	intravenous urography
LBO	large bowel obstruction
LLL	left lower lobe
LOS	lower oesophageal sphincter
LRTI	lower respiratory tract infection
LUL	left upper lobe
LV	left ventricle
LVF	left ventricular failure
MAG3	mercaptoacetyl triglycine
MARS	Medicines (Administration of Radioactive Substances) Regulations
MEN	multiple endocrine neoplasia
MCPJ	metacarpophalangeal joint
MDP	methylene diphosphonate
MR(I)	magnetic resonance (imaging)
MRA	magnetic resonance angiography
MRCP	magnetic resonance cholangiopancreatography
MUGA	multi-gated acquisition
NBM	nil by mouth
Neuro	neurological
NGT	nasogastric tube
NM	nuclear medicine
NSAID	non-steroidal anti-inflammatory drug
NSF	nephrogenic systemic fibrosis
N-STEMI	non-ST elevation myocardial infarction
OA	osteoarthritis
OSCE	Objective Structured Clinical Examination
OGD	oesophagogastroduodenoscopy
OM	occipitomental view
OPG	orthopantomogram
PA	posterior to anterior
PACS	picture archiving and communications system
PCI	percutaneous coronary intervention
PCL	posterior cruciate ligament
PCNL	percutaneous nephrolithotomy
PCS	pelvicalyceal system
PD	proton density
PE	pulmonary embolus
PET	positron emission tomography
PET-CT	combined positron emission tomography with computed tomography
PICC	peripherally inserted central catheter
PIPJ	proximal interphalangeal joint
PT	prothrombin time
PTC	percutaneous transhepatic cholangiography

PUD	peptic ulcer disease
RA	right atrium
RCR	Royal College of Radiologists
RFA	radiofrequency ablation
RLL	right lower lobe
(R)ML	(right) middle lobe
RUL	right upper lobe
RUQ	right upper quadrant
RV	right ventricle
SAH	subarachnoid haemorrhage
SBO	small bowel obstruction
SDH	subdural haemorrhage/haematoma
SIJ	sacroiliac joint
SOL	space occupying lesion
SPECT	single photon emission computed tomography

STEMI	ST elevation myocardial infarction
STIR	short tau inversion recovery
SVC	superior vena cava
TACE	transarterial chemoembolisation
TB	tuberculosis
Tc-99m	metastable technetium-99
TFCC	triangulofibrocartilage complex
TIA	transient ischaemic attack
TIPS	transjugular intrahepatic portosystemic shunt
TNM	tumour, nodes, metastases
UGI	upper gastrointestinal
US	ultrasound
V/Q	ventilation-perfusion
XR	X-ray

Terminology

Attenuation	Gradual loss in intensity of beams and waves including X-rays and ultrasound waves. May also be used synonymously with 'density' to describe appearances on CT imaging (areas of high attenuation are bright whereas areas of low attenuation are dark).
Density	Used synonymously with 'attenuation' to describe appearances on CT imaging (areas of high density are bright whereas areas of low density are dark).
Echogenicity	Used synonymously with 'reflectivity' to describe appearances on ultrasound imaging (hyperechoic areas are bright whereas hypoechoic areas are dark).
Hotspot/Coldspot	Used to describe the uptake of radiopharamaceutical agents by tissues in nuclear medicine imaging (increased uptake results in a hotspot whereas reduced uptake results in a coldspot).

PACS	The 'picture archiving and communication systems' are computer networks that store, retrieve, distribute and present medical images electronically. This permits images to be viewed and manipulated digitally on screen with remote and instant access by multiple users simultaneously and has therefore almost replaced the use of hard-copy films in the UK.
Reflectivity	Used synonymously with 'echogenicity' to describe appearances on ultrasound imaging (hyperreflective areas are bright whereas hyporeflective areas are dark).
Signal	Used to describe appearances on MR imaging (areas of high signal are bright whereas areas of low signal are dark).

1 Plain X-ray (XR) imaging

1.1 The X-ray machine

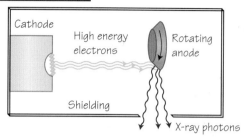

A stream of high energy electrons produced by an electron gun accelerate from a cathode filament and strike a rotating tungsten anode. X-ray photons are generated within the anode which rotates to dissipate heat. The beam of X-ray photons is shielded and coned to reduce the scatter of X-rays produced

1.2 Characteristic radiation generation

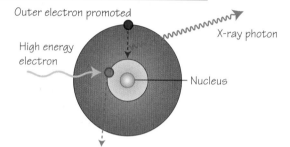

High energy electrons collide with and eject an inner shell tungsten electron (green) with subsequent promotion of an outer shell electron (red) to take its place. X-ray photons of a uniform 'characteristic' energy are generated

1.3 Bremsstrahlung radiation

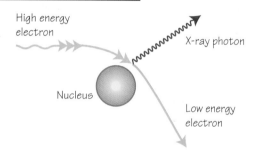

A high energy electron that passes near a tungsten nucleus is deflected and decelerated with generation of an X-ray photon. X-ray photons of variable energy are generated in this way and therefore a non-uniform energy spectrum is produced. This is known as Bremsstrahlung 'Braking' radiation

1.4 The X-ray spectrum

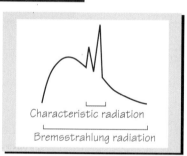

Bremsstrahlung radiation produces a wide spectrum of X-ray energies within the X-ray beam. Characteristic radiation generation however produces a relatively narrow band of X-ray energy. Imaging techniques optimise this characteristic band of X-rays in producing a radiograph

1.5 Image generation

A chest X-ray (CXR) is usually taken with
the beam passing from posterior to anterior (PA).
The X-ray beam is divergent and so the resultant image is magnified.
The closer the patient is to the detector the less magnification is produced.
X-rays which hit the detector uninterrupted appear black on the image. Those X-rays that
pass into thick structures (e.g. heart) or dense structures (e.g. bones) are attenuated and appear white.
Other structures such as the lungs and soft tissues appear as a range of grey, according to their density

Plain XR physics

On 8 November 1895, the German physicist Wilhelm Conrad Röentgen discovered the X-ray, a form of electromagnetic radiation which travels in straight lines at approximately the speed of light. X-rays therefore share the same properties as other forms of electromagnetic radiation and demonstrate characteristics of both waves and particles. X-rays are produced by interactions between accelerated electrons and atoms. When an accelerated electron collides with an atom two outcomes are possible:

1 An accelerated electron displaces an electron from within a shell of the atom. The vacant position left in the shell is filled by an electron from a higher level shell, which results in the release of X-ray photons of uniform energy. This is known as *characteristic radiation.*

2 Accelerated electrons passing near the nucleus of the atom may be deviated from their original course by nuclear forces and thereby transfer some energy into X-ray photons of varying energies. This is known as *Bremsstrahlung radiation.*

The resultant beam of X-ray photons (X-rays) interacts with the body in a number of ways:

• *Absorption* – this prevents the X-rays reaching the X-ray detector plate. Absorption contributes to patient dose and therefore increases the risk of potential harm to the patient.

• *Scatter* – scattering of X-rays is the commonest source of radiation exposure for radiological staff and patients. It also reduces the sharpness of the image.

• *Transmitted* – transmitted X-rays penetrate completely through the body and contribute to the image obtained by causing a uniform blackening of the image.

• *Attenuation* – an X-ray image is composed of transmitted X-rays (black) and X-rays which are attenuated to varying degrees (white to grey). Attenuation can be thought of as a sum of absorption and scatter and is determined by the thickness and density of a structure. In the chest, structures such as the lungs are relatively thick but contain air, making them low in density. The lungs therefore transmit X-rays easily and appear black on the X-ray image. Conversely, bones are not thick but are very dense and therefore appear white. Attenuation can be controlled by varying the power or 'hardness' of the X-ray beam.

The XR machine (tube)

Most modern radiographic machines use electron guns to generate a stream of high energy electrons, which is achieved by heating a filament. The high energy electrons are accelerated towards a target anode. The electrons hit the anode, thereby generating X-rays as described above. This process is very inefficient with 99% of this energy transferred into heat at 60 kV. The dissipation of heat is therefore a key design feature of these machines to sustain their use and maintain their longevity. The material for the target anode is selected depending on the chosen task and the energy of the X-ray beam can be modified by filtration to produce beams of uniform energy.

Most modern radiology departments now employ digital imaging techniques and there are two principal methods in everyday use: computed radiography (CR) and digital radiography (DR). CR uses an exposure plate to create a latent image which is read by a laser stimulating luminescence, before being read by a digital detector. DR systems convert the X-ray image into visible light which is then captured by a photo-voltage sensor that converts the light into electricity, and thus a digital image. The final digital images are stored in medical imaging formats and displayed on computer terminals.

Applying physics to practice

• If the subject to be imaged is placed further from the detector, the image created will be magnified. This is based on the principle that X-ray beams travel in diverging straight lines.

• Scatter from the patient and other objects degrades the resolution. This will cause the image to be blurred.

• Beams of lower energy are absorbed more than beams of higher energy. This affects the difference in clarity between the soft tissue detail and artefact.

Image quality

The clarity of the image can be expressed as 'unsharpness'. This can be classified into:

• *Inherent unsharpness* – this is caused by the structures involved not having sharp, well-defined edges.

• *Movement unsharpness* – this can be reduced by using short exposures, as with light photography.

• *Photographic unsharpness* – this is dependent on the quality and type of imaging equipment and the method of capturing the image. Newer digital imaging systems now allow the post-processing of data to enhance various aspects of the image.

Contrast

The contrast of an image is dependent on the variation of beam attenuation within the subject. There are *five principal densities* that can be seen on a plain radiographic image.

Plain XR densities	
• **Black**	Air/gas
• **Dark grey**	Fat
• **Light grey**	Soft tissue/fluid
• **White**	Bone and calcified structures
• **Bright white**	Metal

The contrast may be increased by lowering the energy of the X-ray beam. However, this has negative impact on image quality and increases the dose of radiation.

Contrast agents are often used to enhance anatomical detail. A desirable contrast agent is one that has high photoelectric absorption at the energy of the X-ray beam. The contrast agents most commonly used in plain X-ray imaging are barium, gastrografin (water soluble) and iodinated compounds. Precautions in the use of iodinated contrast agents are discussed in Chapter 6.

Advantages and disadvantages of plain XR imaging	
Advantages	**Disadvantages**
• Inexpensive	• Radiation exposure
• Fast	• Imaging three-dimensional structures in a two-dimensional format
• Simple	• Low tissue contrast
• Readily available	• Overlapping anatomy
	• No dynamic or functional information

2.1 The image intensifier

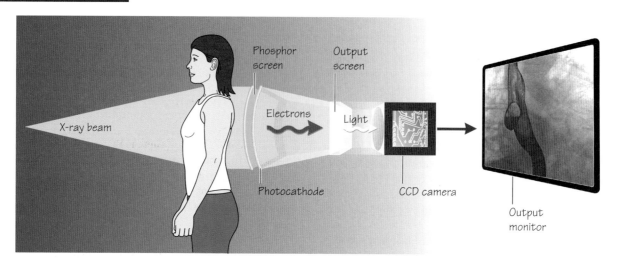

The X-ray beam is directed towards the patient and the image intensifier. The beam strikes the input screen which first contains a phosphor screen. This turns the X-rays into light. This light then strikes the photocathode which generates electrons. These electrons are accelerated and focused onto the output screen, which converts electrons back into a light image. This process intensifies the image brightness by 5000–10,000 times. Digital processing then produces a final image

2.2 Image intensifier overview

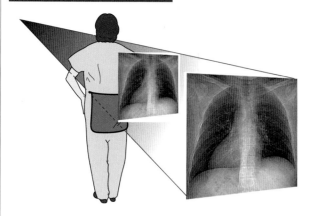

An overview of a body part can be gained without magnification

2.3 Image intensifier magnification

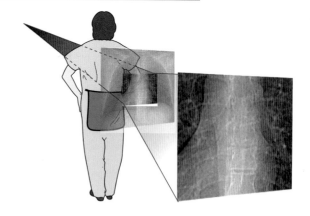

Image intensifiers have a built-in magnification mode that allows 'expansion' of the central portion of the input screen, which fills the output screen to provide magnification of a body part. This means exposing a smaller area of the body to radiation. However, the dose to the body part of interest increases because the X-ray beam intensity is increased in order to maintain the brightness of the image

Principles of fluoroscopy

Fluoroscopy allows dynamic real-time imaging of the patient, which can provide information regarding the movement of anatomical structures or devices within the patient. Fluoroscopy is based on X-ray imaging and the physical principles are similar to the plain X-ray imaging chain from X-ray beam generation to image display (see Chapter 1). However, the procedure is performed using a specifically designed X-ray machine and uses real-time acquisition techniques and hardware.

The fluoroscopy machine

There are two main types of fluoroscopy machines:
- Continuous low energy X-ray production systems.
- Pulsed X-ray production systems – these are used more commonly in practice due to the lower radiation dose given to the patient (and to radiological staff).

Fluoroscopy machines are designed to specifically manage the heat generated from the repeated exposure in fluoroscopic imaging. They also use lower beam energies and exposures compared with plain X-ray imaging techniques and thus *image intensifiers* are employed to enhance the image. These convert the X-rays to electrons to amplify the signal several thousand-fold and then convert the electron beams again into visible light. This light image is then transmitted onto a screen.

Static images, which are similar to plain X-ray images, can be acquired. These provide increased contrast and spatial resolution compared to standard fluoroscopy images, but at the cost of increased patient dose.

Applying physics to practice

When using image intensifiers, several factors must be considered:
- *Patient dose* – this is partially dependent on the distance from the patient to the X-ray tube. It is important to maintain the tube-to-screen distance as large as possible and to place the patient as close as possible to the screen. This will help to keep the doses as low as reasonably achievable (ALARA) (see Chapter 6). The dose is also influenced by the total exposure time and the number of spot images acquired.
- *Image magnification* – the image magnification by the hardware increases the entrance dose to the surface of the patient.
- *Coning* – this reduces the area exposed to radiation therefore reducing the patient dose, but also improves image quality.

Contrast fluoroscopy

For the majority of fluoroscopic imaging, contrast agent enhancement is used. Fluoroscopy gives the ability to make real-time adjustments to the patient's position and image orientation, which often reveals invaluable information to help differentiate the diagnosis. This is most evident when using contrast-enhanced imaging of the bowel.

Applications of fluoroscopy

- **Contrast gastrointestinal imaging**
  - *Videofluoroscopy* – this is a study which takes multiple images per second to look at real-time anatomical and functional properties during the oropharyngeal phase of swallowing.
  - *Contrast swallow* – this is a study looking at real-time images of the anatomical and functional properties of the oesophageal phase of swallowing. This can also give information regarding the oropharyngeal phase but it is less detailed than videofluoroscopy.
  - *Barium meal* – this provides a method of imaging the stomach and proximal small bowel, however it has been largely superseded by endoscopy.
  - *Small bowel meal* – this is a study that provides anatomical and functional information regarding the small bowel. The patient swallows a bolus of contrast agent and then timed interval images are taken as it passes through the small bowel until it reaches the terminal ileum. At this point, focused images are taken to identify diseases of the terminal ileum, e.g. Crohn's disease.
  - *Small bowel enema* – this study is similar to a small bowel meal but contrast agent is pumped through a nasojejunal tube. The bolus is then followed more carefully with real-time images through the entire small bowel. To achieve double contrast, methylcellulose is also given via the nasojejunal tube.
  - *Double contrast barium enema* – this is a study that allows detailed views of the large bowel mucosa. The contrast agent is introduced via a tube per rectum. The patient is then asked to lie in supine, prone and lateral decubitus positions to allow the agent to coat the intraluminal surface of the rectum and large bowel. Gas (air or carbon dioxide) is subsequently pumped via the tube, which inflates the rectum and large bowel, thereby acting as the second (double) contrast agent. Real-time and static images are then taken to map the entire rectum and large bowel. Polyps, cancer and diverticular disease are often detected in this way.
- **ERCP** (endoscopic retrograde cholangiopancreatography) – fluoroscopic imaging with contrast agent is used to perform the cholangiopancreatography aspect of the ERCP procedure in order to delineate the biliary tree.
- **Interventional radiology** – the vast majority of interventional radiology involves fluoroscopy (see Chapter 48).
- **Dynamic cardiac imaging** – anatomical and functional data of heart chambers, valves and coronary arteries.
- **Intraoperative imaging** – one of the commonest applications of intraoperative fluoroscopic imaging is in orthopaedic surgery, where it is used to confirm fracture reduction and positioning of internal fixation devices.

Advantages and disadvantages of fluoroscopy

Advantages	Disadvantages
• Provides dynamic and functional information	• High radiation dose to patient
• Readily available	• Imaging three-dimensional structures in a two-dimensional format
• Inexpensive	• Overlapping anatomy
• Allows real-time interaction	• May be limited by patient mobility and ability to comply

3 Ultrasound (US)

3.1 Ultrasound artefact phenomenon

Ultrasound probe

Hyperechoic object

Acoustic shadowing

Ultrasound wave

Acoustic enhancement

Hypoechoic object

If a sound wave hits a reflective surface such as bone or a calculus, the majority of the wave is reflected back (hyperechoic) and an 'acoustic shadow' is cast. Hypoechoic or anechoic objects such as fluid-filled cysts allow the sound wave to pass with little attenuation. This fools the ultrasound probe's inbuilt compensation, resulting in 'acoustic enhancement' (an artefact that makes the tissue behind the cyst appear bright). Both acoustic shadowing and enhancement are artefacts which can be helpful in image interpretation

3.2 Ultrasound artefact examples

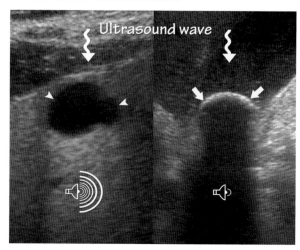

Ultrasound wave

The left image shows a simple hepatic cyst (arrowheads). This is fluid-filled (anechoic) and therefore allows sound to pass freely to the far side of the cyst resulting in 'acoustic enhancement' (loud volume symbol). This artefact can help distinguish a cyst from a solid lesion such as a metastatic deposit. On the right a large gallstone reflects almost all the sound back to the ultrasound probe (hyperechoic). Structures deep to any reflective structure cannot be seen clearly because of the 'acoustic shadow' formed (quiet volume symbol). Gas within the bowel reflects sound in the same way

3.3 The Doppler principle

← Direction of moving object

This picture shows the change in frequency encountered when a source ultrasound beam hits a moving object. If the object is moving towards the source beam (green) the reflected sound beam (red) is 'compressed' and reflected at a higher frequency than the source beam. If however the object is moving away from the source beam then the freqency of the reflected beam (blue) is reduced

3.4 The Doppler principle in practice

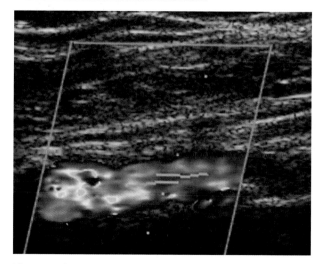

Ultrasound imaging can make use of the Doppler principle in the assessment of blood flow through the cardiovascular system. Here an artery near to a vascular graft is assessed for patency. The red/orange flow represents flow moving predominantly towards the probe

Ultrasound physics

Ultrasound (US) is a dynamic, real-time, imaging modality utilising sound waves in the megahertz range (1–15 MHz), which are completely inaudible to humans. The velocity of sound waves travelling through a medium is dependent on the density of that medium. Sound waves also lose energy to the medium, which is influenced by the wave frequency. This phenomenon is called 'attenuation' and with higher frequencies the attenuation is greater. Consequently high frequency ultrasound is preferable to image superficial structures and low frequency ultrasound is preferable to image deeper structures.

• Image quality
The factors affecting image quality can be split into physics, the machine and the patient. Physics dictates that the image resolution is improved with sound wave beams of shorter wavelength, but the depth of penetration is reduced. Patient factors include bowel gas, depth of adipose tissue, and foreign materials in the beam. Therefore image quality is often compromised in patients with a high body mass index, bowel gas and surgical prostheses in the field of view. Incorrect calibration and usage of the machine can also affect image quality.

• Resolution
The *depth resolution* (clarity in the direction of the sound wave beam) depends on the frequency and length of the ultrasound pulse, and it is approximately half the pulse length. Increasing the frequency, or shortening the beam, increases the depth resolution. *Lateral resolution* (clarity in the direction perpendicular to the direction of the sound wave beam) depends on the width of the beam. Increasing the frequency increases the lateral resolution. However, increasing the frequency reduces the penetration of the beam as it has higher attenuation (as explained above). There is therefore a compromise to be reached between resolution and depth to optimise the imaging.

The US scanner

The ultrasound machine generates and detects ultrasound waves. In addition, it post-processes the returned signals and displays the resultant image.

• Generating and receiving the sound wave
Modern machines use piezo-electric crystal cells to generate and receive ultrasound waves. These materials change dimension in response to an applied electric current. The most popular type is zirconate titanate (PZT). A very short electrical impulse is applied to the crystal-containing transducer, which generates a short pulse at the required resonant frequency. This beam is focused at a specified depth with optimal intensity and lateral resolution for that depth. The beam diverges and is reflected off the surfaces it meets. The reflected beams (echoes) that return to the transducer are also detected by the crystals.

• Creating an image
The image is created by measuring the reflected beams. The signal intensity of the beam is dependent on the distance it has travelled, the object it reflected off, and the characteristics of the media through which it travelled. The effects of attenuation are reduced by boosting the signal from distant objects.

• Probe design
The original design was an 'A-scan' machine that could only plot a single depth point and signal amplitude. The 'B-scan' systems soon followed which can display depth, amplitude and lateral position. Three-dimensional volumetric imaging is currently being introduced and may revolutionise the scope of ultrasound imaging.

• Frame rate
The frame rate is important in imaging moving objects. The electronic systems are limited by information bandwidth and this can adversely affect the image frame rate. The image size, time between pulses, and Doppler applications can also affect the frame rate.

Applications of US

• M-mode
This is a method of imaging moving structures. It images a single point at high frequency to allow visualisation of rapid movement instead of scanning a two-dimensional object. This has traditionally been used in imaging heart valves.

• Doppler imaging
This uses the Doppler effect to calculate velocity. When a sound wave is reflected off a moving object the frequency is modified. If the object is moving towards the receiver, the sound wave is compressed and the frequency rises. If the boundary is moving away from the receiver the opposite is true. Using this phenomenon the velocity of the object can be calculated. Pressure measurements can also be estimated from the Doppler velocity. Doppler imaging is most often used to assess blood flow.

• Continuous and pulsed waved ultrasound
These methods apply the Doppler effect. Continuous wave ultrasound uses two transducers, one to send and one to receive the pulse. Pulsed wave ultrasound uses a single transducer to provide a short signal pulse followed by a period of 'listening' before repeating the signal. This permits attention to be focused on a region of interest by listening at a specific time after the pulse (and therefore specific depth).

• Duplex scanning
This is a combination of Doppler and real-time scanning. The probe collects both sets of data and displays the velocity information in a colour-mapped overlay on the two-dimensional greyscale image.

Contrast US

The use of a contrast agent can enhance the definition of certain tissues and provide additional functional information. In ultrasound the contrast agents currently comprise gas-filled micro-bubbles. These micro-bubbles have a much higher echogenicity compared to surrounding tissues and are useful in assessing blood flow and perfusion.

Advantages and disadvantages of ultrasound

Advantages	Disadvantages
• Relatively inexpensive	• Image quality is dependent on the operator, and patient's body habitus
• Can be portable	
• Not known to be harmful in diagnostic applications (but have the potential to cause burns)	• Limited use in some organ systems, e.g. bone, bowel, lungs
• Good characterisation of solid organs and vascular flow	• Time consuming
• Allows real-time interaction	• Interpretation of static/single images can be difficult

4.1 Third generation CT design

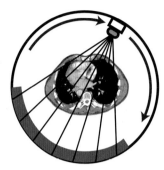

Some scanners still in use are of the third-generation design. The X-ray source and detector array are rigidly fixed to a gantry on either side of the patient. The whole gantry rotates around the patient as the images are taken

4.2 Image creation

The black and white squares within the grid (patient) represent tissues of different densities. At each point on the axial rotation an image is taken of the tissue slice. These images are then transferred to a computer where powerful mathematics is used to produce a final image of the tissue slice

4.3 Multislice helical scanning

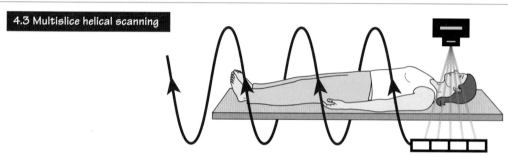

In modern multiple-slice CT scanner design an array of detectors captures multiple 'slices' of anatomy in a single acquisition. The X-ray source and the detector array form a unit which rotates around the patient as the CT table moves through the bore of the scanner. The imaging data is therefore essentially acquired in a 'helix'. The most recent generation of scanners have several hundred detectors and use lower doses to acquire large volumes of imaging data with each rotation and with reduced artefact from patient movement

4.4 Hounsfield units (HU)

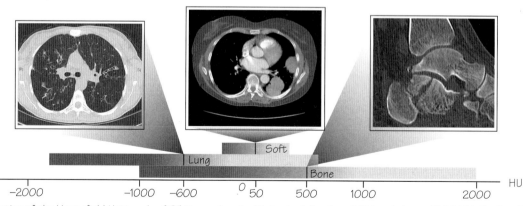

This is a representation of the Hounsfield Unit scale of CT tissue density. Water is defined as 0 HU and air as -1000 HU. The 'level' is the HU (density) at the centre of the 'window' and is positioned to optimise detail of particular tissues within the anatomical region imaged. The 'window' is the range of units that are displayed within the image greyscale either side of the 'level'. Outside this range the values are shown as black if of lower density or white if of higher density. Example 'levels' and 'windows' are shown: 'soft tissue windows' (L = 50, W = 300); 'lung windows' (L = -600, W = 1200); and 'bone windows' (L = 500, W = 1500)

Computed tomography physics

Modern computed tomography (CT) was invented by the English electrical engineer, Sir Godfrey Hounsfield, in 1967 and since then has revolutionised radiology and medical practice as a whole. The physics of CT is based on generating a three-dimensional image from multiplanar two-dimensional X-ray images taken around the craniocaudal axis. The premise for the technique is based on the predictability of X-ray attenuation within different materials due to each material's individual electron density and atomic number. Plain X-ray imaging is hampered by the overlapping of anatomical structures, which reduces the contrast range and obscures anatomical information. CT, however, can provide:
- Improved contrast resolution.
- Improved structural definition.
- The ability to digitally manipulate acquired images.

CT achieves this by attempting to view the same structure from many angles and thereby provides a number of dimensions to extrapolate an object's image density. In modern CT machines the X-ray tube rotates around the patient, exposing only a thin axial slice of the body to X-rays from multiple angles. The axial slice is divided into a grid of small voxels (three-dimensional pixels) and the attenuation of each voxel is calculated to reconstruct the final image. This is performed for every voxel on every slice to generate a series of images. The resultant image benefits from:
- Improved range of image contrast (over 4000 levels compared to the five of plain X-ray imaging).
- Three-dimensional imaging (allows the separation of anatomical structures).
- Various post-processing algorithms (highlight features of interest).
- Isometric data (allows reconstruction of images, which can be manipulated after acquisition, e.g. 'reformatting' in any desired plane and 'rendering' to demonstrate surfaces. The images can then be rotated, panned and magnified to aid interpretation).

The use of multi-slice X-rays in CT imaging exposes the patient to significantly higher doses of radiation compared with plain X-ray imaging. For example, an abdominal CT gives a dose of 10 mSv compared to 1 mSv from a plain AXR.

Hounsfield units (HU)

The Hounsfield unit scale is used to calibrate the greyscale applied to the X-ray attenuation of the materials in every image. This is defined with water density being 0 HU and air −1000 HU. Bone is in the order of +1000 HU. The image can be manipulated by changing certain Hounsfield unit variables to accentuate or focus on certain tissues within an image. This is known as 'windowing' and 'levelling'.
- *Windowing* – only a preselected range of Hounsfield units is displayed. If the 'window' width is reduced, a narrower range of Hounsfield unit values are displayed across the same number of pixels. In this way, smaller differences in attenuation can be appreciated.

- *Levelling* – this is the level around which the 'window' is preset and allows finer detail in specific tissues to be appreciated (centre of window).

The CT scanner

Since the advent of CT imaging there have been several generations of scanner design. The current multislice CT scanners involve a single X-ray tube opposite multiple rows of detectors that axially rotate around the patient. The array of detectors is the most important component of the machine as this is where the images are acquired. The array is created by a matrix of multiple detector banks arranged in parallel rows. The number of slices, for example a '64-slice scanner', indicates the number of concurrent tissue slices the rows of detectors are able to image. Increasing the slice thickness allows a larger amount of tissue to be scanned per revolution and may be used when imaging the beating heart, for example. The current generation of scanners can acquire images in a few seconds.

Applications of CT

There are many applications of CT technology and these are constantly expanding. Many of these different applications vary by their software profiles whereas the basic hardware is often identical. Common applications include:
- *Diagnostic CT imaging* – CT can be used for diagnostic purposes in all regions of the body.
- *CT angiography* – contrast agent enhanced CT imaging of vessels can clearly reveal vascular pathology. Further post-processing can render the vessels for even easier visualisation.
- *Cardiac CT* – this is often performed using 'ECG-gated' scanning, whereby slices of the heart are imaged at the identical point in the cardiac cycle. This allows an accurate composite image to be created of a constantly moving object. Newer and more advanced CT imaging technology is emerging which may soon supersede the need for ECG-gating.
- *CT fluoroscopy* – this allows real-time dynamic imaging using CT and is used in interventions and biopsies.

Contrast agents

Contrast agents greatly add to the diagnostic value in CT imaging. There are many types of contrast agents routinely used but the commonest include iodinated intravascular agents, which resolve vascular and well-perfused structures. A 'negative' oral contrast agent, e.g. water, is commonly used for stomach and proximal small bowel imaging studies. For large bowel imaging studies, a 'positive' contrast agent, e.g. dilute barium sulphate, is usually used. Gas in the form of air or carbon dioxide can also be administered rectally to provide double-contrast imaging. CT imaging of the abdomen is however contraindicated for several days after a conventional barium enema due to the artefact encountered by the dense barium contrast agent.

Advantages and disadvantages of CT

Advantages
- Excellent contrast range
- Excellent anatomical definition
- Isometric volume dataset allows three-dimensional reconstruction
- Fast scan times (ideal for emergency cases)

Disadvantages
- High radiation dose
- Soft tissue definition is not as good as MRI
- Expensive

5 Magnetic resonance imaging (MRI)

5.1 T1 relaxation

a

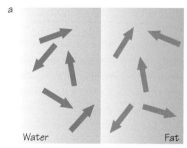

Water   Fat

b

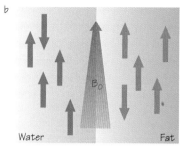

Water   Fat

c

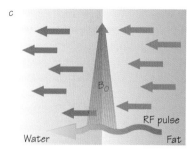

RF pulse

Water   Fat

d

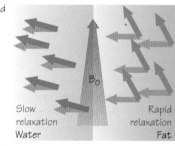

Slow relaxation Water   Rapid relaxation Fat

The body's hydrogen nuclei behave as 'bar magnets' which are randomly aligned (a). When an external magnetic field 'B₀' is applied to the body the magnetic vectors of most hydrogen nuclei line up along the field lines of B_O (b). When an RF pulse is then applied these vectors are tipped into a transverse plane (c). When this RF pulse is removed the vectors 'relax' to their initial longitudinal position (d). Detection of T1 MR signal occurs during this relaxation process and the final MR image comprises a graphic representation of differences in T1 characteristics of tissues. Hydrogen nuclei within tissues predominantly containing fat relax rapidly and produce high T1 signal, which is a measure of the return of hydrogen nuclei from transverse to longitudinal axis alignment. Fat therefore appears bright on T1-weighted images. Hydrogen nuclei within tissues predominantly containing water relax more slowly and produce a low T1 signal and therefore appear dark on T1-weighted images

5.2 T2 relaxation

a

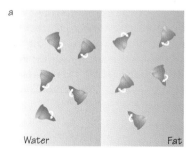

Water   Fat

b

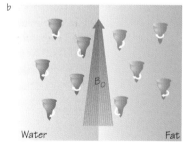

Water   Fat

c

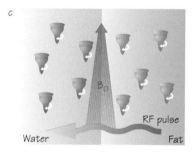

RF pulse

Water   Fat

d

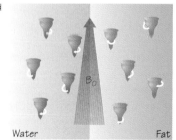

Water   Fat

The body's hydrogen nuclei are randomly aligned and are 'spinning' on their own axis (a). When an external magnetic field 'B₀' is applied to the body (b) the nuclei align (as in Fig 5.1b) but also 'precess' (spin around their axis at a specific frequency related to the energy of B_O). When an RF pulse is then applied (c) the spinning nuclei are forced into 'phase' (coherent synchronised spinning). When this RF pulse is removed however, the nuclei lose this phase coherence and 'relax' to return to their random phases (d). Detection of T2 MR signal tissue contrast occurs during this dephasing process and the final MR image comprises a graphic representation of differences in T2 characteristics of tissues. Hydrogen nuclei within tissues predominantly containing water dephase slowly and maintain high T2 signal. Water therefore appears bright on T2-weighted images. Hydrogen nuclei within tissues predominantly containing fat dephase more rapidly and therefore lose T2 signal. Fat is therefore less bright than water on T2-weighted images

Magnetic resonance physics

Magnetic resonance imaging (MRI) is an advanced imaging technique that uses magnetic fields in place of radiation to generate images. MRI works by manipulating the natural magnetic properties of hydrogen nuclei, which are essentially protons and present in abundance throughout body tissues. Each hydrogen nucleus spins on its own axis, generating an individual magnetic field and so the entire body can be thought to contain multiple tiny randomly aligned bar magnets. When an external magnetic field ('B_0') is applied to the body these bar magnets line up with the field lines of B_0. Some spinning hydrogen nuclei line up in the opposite direction, however, the net magnetic vector is in line with B_0. The B_0 field also causes the hydrogen nuclei to spin on their axes at a specific frequency. This is called 'precession'. If a radiofrequency energy pulse (RF pulse) is then applied the aligned magnetic vectors are tipped into the x-y plane and the spins of the hydrogen nuclei synchronise to gain 'phase coherence'. When the RF pulse is switched off the hydrogen nuclei begin to 'relax' by releasing RF energy. This phenomenon is ultimately responsible for image production and comprises several important processes:

• The spinning hydrogen nuclei are again only subject to B_0 and begin 'relaxing' to align with the B_0 field lines. This is *T1 relaxation* or spin-lattice relaxation.

• The spinning hydrogen nuclei begin to desynchronise and lose phase coherence. This is *T2 relaxation* (also known as spin-spin relaxation because of the interactions between the spinning hydrogen nuclei and their individual magnetic fields).

• The strength of the B_0 field is not completely uniform and some spinning hydrogen nuclei are subject to slightly stronger magnetic field forces than others. This affects the pattern of loss of phase coherence of the spins and is known as *T2* (T2 star) relaxation*.

When hydrogen nuclei are spinning with phase coherence a current is induced in the receiver coil, creating a signal that can be processed into an image pixel. As hydrogen nuclei lose phase coherence there is reduced current induction and signal strength decreases. Since different tissues have different densities of spinning hydrogen nuclei, their relaxation times vary. This creates signal differentiation on the image.

Light molecules, such as free water, are less effective in losing their energy and therefore have longer T1 and T2 relaxation times. Heavier molecules, such as fat or protein, are more effective at losing their energy and therefore have shorter T1 and T2 relaxation times. Both water and fat have fast T2* relaxation times.

To map a signal to a specific position and orientation within the body, further magnetic field gradients need to be applied. This generates complex data to allow the exact position within the body to be plotted.

Sequences

Different tissue types have different image characteristics due to their T1 and T2 relaxation times. MR imaging techniques are therefore manipulated in many ways to create optimal image sequences for the structures of interest. This process is known as 'weighting' and is achieved by adjusting multiple variables including the RF pulse magnitude and the time between consecutive RF pulses. The sequences that are most commonly used include:

• *T1-weighted (T1-W)* – excellent for imaging anatomy.
• *T2-weighted (T2-W)* – excellent for imaging pathology.
• *Proton density (PD)* – excellent for both anatomy and pathology.
• *Fat saturation* – the signal from fat is suppressed. It is most commonly used with contrast-enhanced imaging and to highlight structures on T1-weighted imaging.
• *Short-tau inversion recovery (STIR)* – this sequence nulls the signal from fat more effectively than fat saturation and is excellent at visualising fluid such as bone oedema.

The MR scanner

Conventional MR machines have a narrow aperture for the patient and can cause problems with claustrophobic and obese patients. The B_0 magnetic field is usually provided by a superconducting magnet which is permanently active, giving a field of 0.2–3 tesla in modern machines. The RF pulses and gradient magnetic fields are generated by perpendicular magnets, which are only active during the scan and recognised by their loud clicking noise. Due to the constantly active superconducting magnet, the MR suite is classed as a restricted area for health and safety reasons. All attenders to the scanner room (except for the patient) must be qualified to enter. This is the only area in a hospital where cardiopulmonary resuscitation cannot be performed due to the hazards of the strong magnetic field and must therefore be performed outside the scanner room.

Applications of MR (see Chapter 42 for contraindications)

There are numerous applications of MR:

• Basic MR imaging is performed with and without a contrast agent to look for pathology including tumours and infection.
• MR arthrograms are performed with a contrast agent injected into a joint, enhancing soft tissue definition of anatomical structures.
• MR angiography is based on the principle that moving magnetised blood will have left the frame of reference by the time the signal is measured. This gives vessels a negative (black) signal on conventional sequences and results in its own contrast phenomenon.

Contrast agents (see Chapter 6 for precautions)

In most applications, innate tissue contrast is adequate for image interpretation. However, when greater clarity and detail or functional imaging is required, a contrast agent can be used, which may be administered intravenously or intra-articularly. Gadolinium is a paramagnetic metal ion agent that alters local tissue magnetism, adding contrast to the image.

Advantages and disadvantages of MRI

Advantages	Disadvantages
• No radiation exposure	• Lengthy scanning times and expensive
• Excellent for imaging soft tissues	• Most MR imaging is still not three-dimensional
• Multi-planar imaging	• Can be technically difficult to perform and interpret
• Functional imaging, e.g. perfusion, diffusion	• Contraindicated in patients with a pacemaker, defibrillator
• Metabolic imaging by using MR spectroscopy	device, hearing aid, cochlear implant

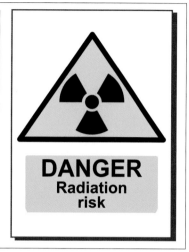

6.1 Radiation protection: principles and legislation

- ALARA — As Low As Reasonably Achievable
- IRR99 — protecting the employee in the workplace
- IR(ME)R — protecting the patient during investigation and treatment
- MARS regulations 1978 — license to administer radioactive medicines

6.2 Contrast agent risks

- Iodinated contrast agents: Hypersensitivity reactions, contrast induced nephropathy (in patients with renal impairment)
- Gadolinium: Nephrogenic systemic fibrosis (in patients with renal impairment)

DANGER
Radiation risk

Radiation exposure

Radiation does not stimulate any of the human senses and therefore exposure is silent. The consequences of radiation exposure may be irreversible and even lethal. The adverse effects of radiation exposure include:

- *Deterministic effects* – these are directly related to the dose of radiation to which the individual is exposed and can vary from simple erythema to significant cell damage and death. Beyond certain threshold levels, cells that are actively engaged in the cell cycle are targeted, resulting typically in bone marrow suppression and gastrointestinal side effects.
- *Stochastic effects* – these are predicted from the probability of occurrence. Their severity however is not dose related and hence there is no threshold level. The majority of *carcinogenic* and *genetic effects* of radiation exposure for medical purposes fall into this category.

Radiation protection

The principles of radiation protection are:

- *Justification* – the purpose for conducting the examination should justify the radiation exposure.
- *Optimisation* – the dose should be *as low as reasonably achievable* (ALARA) to ensure an adequate examination.
- *Dose limitation* – radiographers should record the dose given to each patient to help ensure dose limitation.

Radiation legislation

Protecting patients and medical staff from the harmful effects of radiation is ensured by UK legislation. Imaging Departments and other areas using ionising radiation are regularly investigated and audited to maintain stringent safe practice.

Ionising Radiation Regulations 1999 (IRR99)

The Health and Safety Executive (HSE) is responsible for IRR99. The aim of this legislation is to *protect the employee and general public from ionising radiation in the workplace*. IRR99 defines the responsibilities of the:

- *Employer* – to perform risk assessment, authorise practices and liaise with the HSE.
- *Employee* – to work within the defined practices, report failures, look after their own equipment and not knowingly overexpose themselves or other employees.

Dose limits for employees are defined together with the designation of *controlled* and *supervised* areas which are determined by the level of predicted exposure.

Ionising Radiation (Medical Exposure) Regulations 2000 – IR(ME)R

The Department of Health is responsible for IR(ME)R. The aim of this legislation is to *protect patients undergoing medical examinations and treatments with ionising radiation*. IR(ME)R defines various roles and responsibilities.

- *Employer* (e.g. the hospital) – must provide a framework for employees.
- *Referrer* (e.g. the referring clinician) – must provide adequate and correct information to allow justification of the examination.
- *Practitioner* (usually the radiologist) – decides the appropriate imaging and justifies the exposure.
- *Operator* (the radiologist or radiographer) – authorises and performs the exposure with dose optimisation.

Protocols must be written in each Radiology/Imaging Department for all radiological procedures and for each piece of equipment, as well as giving a reference dose level. A written framework must be created for procedures, maintenance, quality assurance and audit.

Medicines (Administration of Radioactive Substances) Regulations 1978 – MARS regulations 1978

The Administration of Radioactive Substances Advisory Committee (ARSAC) is responsible for the MARS regulations 1978. This legislation requires doctors who administer radioactive medicines to humans to hold a licence to do so.

Iodinated contrast agent precautions

Many X-ray imaging investigations, especially CT, use intravenous iodinated contrast agents to obtain greater diagnostic information, for example, delineating the inner structure of vessels and detecting pathological processes including malignancy and infection. In addition, the vascular supply to organs can be ascertained. The benefits of using an iodinated contrast agent however must be weighed against the risk of its potential adverse effects along with the risk of radiation exposure. In some circumstances, an imaging study that does not use a contrast agent or radiation may answer the question. The potential adverse effects of administering an iodinated contrast agent can be divided into general, CIN and thyrotoxicosis.

General adverse reactions

Iodinated contrast agents may cause hypersensitivity reactions in susceptible individuals, e.g. asthmatics, patients with other drug allergies, and patients who have suffered previous adverse reactions. The hypersensitivity reactions may manifest as:
- *Immediate IgE-mediated hypersensitivity reaction* – occurs within an hour of administration of the contrast agent and can range from urticaria to a major anaphylactoid reaction.
- *Delayed T-cell mediated hypersensitivity reaction* – occurs later than one hour following administration of the contrast agent and usually causes erythematous skin rashes.

It is important to note that a patient with a previous delayed hypersensitivity reaction is not at increased risk of an immediate hypersensitivity reaction, and vice versa, due to the different immunological processes.

Patients who develop adverse contrast agent hypersensitivity reactions should be managed according to the severity of the symptoms. Severe reactions must be treated as a *medical emergency* and may require immediate resuscitation with oxygen therapy, intravenous fluids and treatment with a bronchodilator, antihistamine and adrenaline.

Contrast-induced nephropathy (CIN)

CIN is defined as acute renal impairment that occurs within three days of administration of an intravascular contrast agent without any other identifiable cause. It is one of the commonest causes of hospital-acquired acute renal failure and is thought to be due to renal ischaemia and direct toxic effects on the renal tubular epithelium. Patients at highest risk are those with pre-existing renal impairment such as those with diabetes mellitus or taking nephrotoxic drugs. Preventive measures should therefore be taken in patients with moderate or severe renal impairment, which is often based on their estimated glomerular filtration rate (eGFR):

Normal renal function	eGFR above 90 ml/min/1.73 m^2
Mild renal impairment	eGFR 61–89 ml/min/1.73 m^2
Moderate renal impairment	eGFR below 60 ml/min/1.73 m^2
Severe renal impairment	eGFR below 30 m/min/1.73 m^2

Precautionary measures include:
- Considering *alternative investigations*.
- *Withholding nephrotoxic drugs*, e.g. metformin for 48 hours post-administration and rechecking the renal function before restarting.
- *Oral hydration* (100 ml/hour for four hours) prior to administration and 24 hours post-administration is strongly recommended in patients with moderate renal impairment.
- *Intravenous hydration* (100 ml/hour for 4 hours) prior and 24 hours post-administration is strongly recommended in patients with severe renal impairment. Hydration is thought to reduce the risk of renal ischaemia and dilute the contrast agent in the renal tubules.
- *Rechecking renal function* 48–72 hours post-administration.

Thyrotoxicosis

Patients with hyperthyroidism should not be given iodinated contrast agents as they are at high risk of developing thyrotoxicosis post-administration. Patients with thyroid disease including Grave's disease, multinodular goitre and thyroid autonomy are also at risk but may be given an iodinated contrast agent if they are closely monitored by an endocrinologist post-administration.

MR contrast agent precautions

The most commonly used contrast agent in MR scanning is gadolinium. Its safety is still under assessment and several cases of *nephrogenic systemic fibrosis (NSF)* following exposure to gadolinium have been reported in patients with *pre-existing renal impairment*. NSF is a severe syndrome characterised by fibrosis of the skin, eyes, joints, muscles, liver, lungs and heart. The use of gadolinium must therefore be used with caution in patients with pre-existing renal impairment.

Risk of fatal cancer from medical radiation

CXR (0.02–0.06 mSv) Extremity XR (0.01 mSv)	1 in 500,000–1,000,000
AXR (1 mSv) Hip and pelvis XR (0.7 mSv) Lumbar spine XR (1 mSv) CT head (2 mSv)	1 in 10,000–100,000
IVU (1.5 mSv) Barium swallow/meal (2 mSv) Barium enema (4 mSv) CT chest (8 mSV) CT abdomen (10 mSV) CT spine (10 mSv) CT cardiac (20 mSv)	1 in 1000–10,000

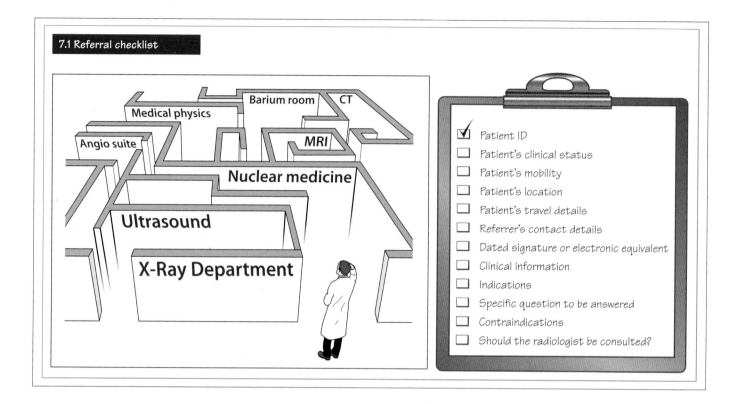

7.1 Referral checklist

Medical physics · Barium room · CT · Angio suite · MRI · Nuclear medicine · Ultrasound · X-Ray Department

Checklist:
- ☑ Patient ID
- ☐ Patient's clinical status
- ☐ Patient's mobility
- ☐ Patient's location
- ☐ Patient's travel details
- ☐ Referrer's contact details
- ☐ Dated signature or electronic equivalent
- ☐ Clinical information
- ☐ Indications
- ☐ Specific question to be answered
- ☐ Contraindications
- ☐ Should the radiologist be consulted?

Optimising the referral request

The Imaging Department is integral to the multidisciplinary team managing a patient's care. The referrer should therefore aim to involve the Imaging Department early in the care of appropriate patients. The following are useful pointers to get the most from the Imaging Department:
- Make early referrals, e.g. immediately after the ward round when the decision for an imaging referral has been made, thereby ensuring the Imaging Department can manage the referral request promptly and efficiently.
- The referrer must be familiar with the indications for investigation and have a specific question to be answered by the investigation when making the referral or when discussing with the radiographer or radiologist.
- The referrer must have considered the contraindications and risks related to radiation and iodinated intravenous contrast agents before making the referral.
- Multidisciplinary team meetings are useful forums to gain comprehensive feedback from the radiologists on referred cases.
- Radiologists are often very broadly experienced clinicians and can therefore offer a wide-ranging expert opinion on diagnosis and management when consulted appropriately.

The radiology referral request

The referral request form is a legal document, whether in paper or electronic format. The referrer carries the responsibility to ensure that the correct and complete information is conveyed to the Imaging Department so that patients are appropriately diagnosed and managed.

The core information that must be communicated includes:
- **Patient identification details:** The most important point on any checklist is checking that the correct patient receives the correct investigation or procedure. The referrer must ensure that the Imaging Department receives the correct identification details of the patient to be investigated. The essentials are:
  - *full name*
  - *date of birth*
  - *hospital identification number.*
- **Clinical status:** The referrer must convey the patient's clinical condition and urgency of the referral to the Imaging Department. If there is doubt the referrer should consult the radiologist.
- **Patient mobility:** The referrer must always consider the patient's mobility and compliance for the desired imaging investigation before making the referral. For example, a request for a barium enema is inappropriate if the patient is immobile, as this investigation involves rolling over on the X-ray table.
- **Patient location and travel details:** The patient's mobility also extends to their mode of transport to the Imaging Department. This includes the need for a clinical escort with patients requiring monitoring and therapeutic adjuncts, e.g. supplementary oxygen and intravenous infusions. The points of departure, return and contact details must also be notified to the Imaging Department to ensure the patient is transferred safely and efficiently. For outpatient referrals consideration must be given to the patient's ability to attend without support.
- **Referrer contact details:** While filling in a referral form it is vital to complete the referrer's contact details in case any further informa-

tion needs to be directly communicated. A named responsible consultant is also required to ensure the report is logged and forwarded to the correct clinical team.

• **Dated signature (or electronic equivalent):** This is mandatory, without which the investigation will not be performed.

• **Clinical information:** This section of the referral request should be completed with care. The information must include sufficient detail to allow the reporting radiologist to appreciate the specific clinical problem in question. It should also provide adequate clinical appropriateness to justify the use of expensive resources and to warrant exposure to ionising radiation in investigations using X-rays. Both the indications and contraindications should be considered for each investigation in every patient.

• **Indications:** Interpretation of imaging investigations should never be independent of the overall clinical setting. Indications for referral must therefore include salient features of the current clinical problem:

  ○ *presenting complaint*
  ○ *past medical and surgical history (and gynaecological history in females)*
  ○ *relevant physical examination findings*
  ○ *results of other relevant investigations*
  ○ *results of relevant previous imaging*
  ○ *The referral indication should also include a specific question to be answered by the imaging investigation.*

The referrer is often unsure as to the most appropriate imaging investigation for the clinical problem and so it is good practice to discuss the clinical problem and differential diagnosis with the radiologist performing the procedure. The radiologist can then offer an expert opinion and helpful guidance.

• **Contraindications:** Many imaging modalities expose the patient to ionising radiation and the referrer must therefore always consider the risk of harm against the likely benefit of a specific investigation. The Royal College of Radiologists defines a 'useful investigation' as one in which the result, positive or negative, will inform clinical management and/or add confidence to the clinician's diagnosis.[1] Wasteful use of radiology includes *repeating investigations already performed, performing investigations which are unlikely to alter patient management, investigating too early, doing the wrong investigation, failing to ask an appropriate clinical question that the imaging investigation should answer, and over-investigating.* Other factors to also consider include:

  ○ In investigations involving radiation exposure to the female pelvis, a *history of the last menstrual period must be taken in those of reproductive age* to ensure a pregnant pelvis is not unknowingly irradiated.
  ○ Intravenous contrast agents are nephrotoxic and thus the *renal function status* must be reviewed prior to their use. Many Imaging Departments now insist on having details of up-to-date renal function test results included on the referral form if an intravenous contrast agent is likely to be used. Furthermore, patients must have appropriate untravenous access.
  ○ *Ferromagnetic implants and foreign bodies are contraindicated for MR imaging.* Pacemakers are considered a contraindication due to the risk of malfunction. Other contraindications include hearing aids and cochlear implants.
  ○ Needles are used in interventional radiology procedures and thus the patient's *coagulation status* must be checked before the procedure and the results conveyed to the Imaging Department.

If there is any ongoing doubt and the situation is not an emergency, the referrer should delay the investigation, consider an alternative investigation, or consult the radiologist.

[1] The Royal College of Radiologists. *Making the best use of clinical radiology services: referral guidelines.* London: The Royal College of Radiologists, 2007. Available via the College website (http://www.rcr.ac.uk).

Which investigation: classic cases

Trauma scenarios

Clinical case	Primary test	Other tests
ATLS protocol*	C-spine XR, CXR, pelvis XR	CT neck, chest, abdomen, pelvis
Head injury	CT head[†]	
Orbital trauma	XR face, orbits	CT
Facial trauma	XR face	CT
Mandibular trauma	XR mandible, OPG	
Spinal injury	XR (pain)	CT (MR if neuro deficit)
Fall and unable to weight-bear	XR pelvis + lateral hip	CT, MR
Simple pneumothorax	CXR	CT
Abdominal injury	Erect CXR + AXR	CT
Renal trauma	CT	IVU, US
Limb injury	XR	CT, MR, US
Scaphoid #	4-view XR	MR, CT
Foreign body	XR	US

*Advanced Trauma Life Support. American College of Surgeons 2008
[†]Head Injury. Methods, Evidence & Guidance. NICE 2007

Gastrointestinal scenarios

Clinical case	Primary test	Other tests
Dysphagia	Ba swallow	Videofluoroscopy
UGI anastamotic leak	Contrast swallow, meal	
Abdominal pain	AXR	US, CT
Obstruction, perforation	Erect CXR + AXR	CT
Change in bowel habit	Colonoscopy, Ba enema	CT, CT colonography
IBD (exacerbation)	AXR	CT, MR, NM
IBD (chronic)	Colonoscopy	Ba enema, CT colonoscopy
Abdominal mass	US	CT
Abdominal sepsis	US	CT
Liver metastases	US, CT	MR, PET-CT
Cirrhosis	US	CT, MR
Jaundice	US	ERCP, CT, MRCP, PTC, EndoUS
Biliary leak	US	MRCP, NM

Cardiovascular and respiratory scenarios

Clinical case	Primary test	Other tests
STEMI	CXR, PCI	Echo, CT, MR, NM
N-STEMI	CXR, Echo	CTA, MR, NM
Heart failure	CXR, Echo	MR, CT, NM
PE	CXR	CTPA, NM, MRA
AAA	US	CT, MR, CTA
Ischaemic leg	Duplex US	CTA, MRA, Angiography
DVT	Duplex US	Venography
LRTI	CXR	
Pleural effusion	CXR	US, CT
Haemoptysis	CXR	CT, Angiography

ENT scenarios

Clinical case	Primary test	Other tests
Middle ear symptoms	CT, MR	
Sensorineural hearing loss	MR	
Sinus disease	CT	
Neck lump	US	CT, MR
Thyroid disease	US	FNAC, NM
Salivary duct obstruction	US, Sialogram	

Musculoskeletal scenarios

Clinical case	Primary test	Other tests
Atlanto-axial subluxation	XR (flexion + extension)	CT, MR
Back pain	XR,[‡] MR	CT, NM
?Osteomyelitis	XR	MR, CT, NM
Bone/joint pain	XR	MR, CT, NM
Bone metastasis	XR, MR	NM
Soft tissue mass	XR, US, MR	
Myeloma	XR skeletal survey	MRI
Metabolic bone disease	XR	DEXA, NM
Arthropathy	XR joint	XR hands + feet, US, MR, NM

[‡]in specific circumstances only (see Chapter 46)

Head and neurological scenarios

Clinical case	Primary test	Other tests
Stroke	CT	MR, CTA, Carotid US
TIA	CT, carotid US	Angiography, CTA, MRA
Intracranial mass	CT, MR	
Sudden, severe headache	CT	MR, CTA
Posterior fossa signs	CT, MR	
Dementia	CT, MR	NM
?Venous sinus thrombosis	CT, MR	CT, MR venography

Genitourinary and gynaecological scenarios

Clinical case	Primary test	Other tests
Renal failure	AXR, US	CT, MR, NM
Renal colic	CT KUB, IVU	
Renal mass	Renal tract US	CT, MR
Microscopic haematuria	KUB + Renal tract US	
Macroscopic haematuria	KUB + Renal tract US, cystoscopy	IVU, CT urography
Prostatism	Pelvic US	
Scrotal mass, pain	Testicular US	
Postmenopausal bleeding	Pelvic US	
Unresponsive hypertension	Renal MRA	Renal artery US, CTA

Cancer scenarios

Cancer	Diagnosis	Staging
Oropharynx, larynx	CT, MR	CT, MR, US, PET-CT
Parotid	US, MR, CT	CT, MR, PET-CT
Thyroid	US, NM	CT, MR, US, NM
Lung	CXR, CT	CT, PET-CT
Oesophagus	Ba swallow, Endoscopy	CT, EndoUS, PET-CT
Stomach	OGD, Ba meal	CT
Liver primary	US, MR, CT	MR, CT
Liver secondary	US, MR, CT, PET-CT	
Pancreas	US, CT, MR, MRCP	US, CT, MR, PET-CT

Cancer	Diagnosis	Staging
Colon/rectum	Ba enema, CT colonography, colonoscopy	CXR, US, CT, MR, PET-CT
Kidney	US, CT	CXR, CT, MR, PET-CT
Bladder	US, IVU	CXR, CT, MR, IVU, PET-CT
Prostate	US	MR, NM
Testicle	US	CT
Ovary	US, MR	CT, MR, PET-CT
Uterus	US, MR	MR
Cervix	MR	CT, MR, PET-CT
Lymphoma	US, CT	CT, MR, PET-CT
Bone/soft tissue	XR, US, CT, MR, NM	CT, MR, PET-CT

The Royal College of Radiologists produces evidence-based guidelines for referrers to determine the most appropriate imaging investigation for a wide range of clinical problems. Appropriate investigations are those that inform clinical management and/or add confidence to the clinical diagnosis. It is important to note that not every patient in each clinical scenario will require an imaging investigation and indeed in many cases one of the 'other tests' may be more appropriate as the primary test of choice. The information presented here is adapted from the RCR guidelines to provide an overview to assist in constructing the most appropriate imaging strategies. The RCR guidelines should be consulted for more complete details.[1]

[1] The Royal College of Radiologists. *Making the best use of clinical radiology services: referral guidelines*. London: The Royal College of Radiologists, 2007. Available via the College website (http://www.rcr.ac.uk).

9.1 CXR referral checklist

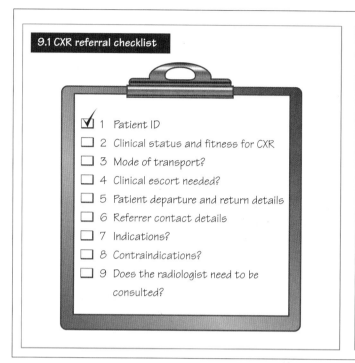

☑ 1 Patient ID

☐ 2 Clinical status and fitness for CXR

☐ 3 Mode of transport?

☐ 4 Clinical escort needed?

☐ 5 Patient departure and return details

☐ 6 Referrer contact details

☐ 7 Indications?

☐ 8 Contraindications?

☐ 9 Does the radiologist need to be
consulted?

9.2 Approach to CXR interpretation

1 Image ID

2 Patient ID

3 Technical adequacy

4 Artefacts and foreign bodies

5 Trachea

6 Lungs

7 Heart

8 Mediastinum

9 Hila

10 Hemidiaphragms

11 Review areas –
costophrenic angles,
apices, behind heart
and under the diaphragm,
bones, soft tissues

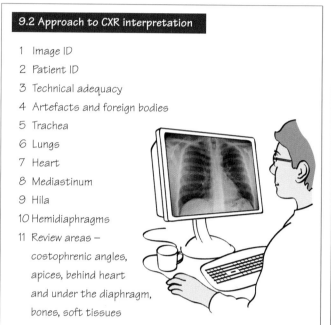

CXR referral checklist (see Chapter 7)

The imaging referral form is a legal document. The referrer carries the responsibility to ensure the correct and complete information is conveyed to the Imaging Department so that the patient is appropriately diagnosed and managed.

• **Patient identification:** The referrer must ensure that the Imaging Department receives the correct identification details of the patient to be investigated: full name, date of birth, and hospital identification number are the essentials.

• **Clinical status:** The referrer must convey the patient's clinical condition and urgency of the referral to the Imaging Department. A CXR is commonly the first-line investigation for acute cardiorespiratory complaints or in the monitoring of chronic chest conditions; however, in some circumstances alternative imaging may be more appropriate, e.g. CT or MRI. If there is doubt the referrer should consult the radiologist.

• **Patient mobility:** Optimal images are obtained with the patient in deep inspiration. Incomplete inspiration compromises the information that can be obtained from the image, e.g. the heart appears artificially enlarged (pseudocardiomegaly). The ideal projection for a CXR is PA sitting or preferably standing. The patient must be able to hold themselves upright but, if they cannot, a departmental or mobile AP image can be obtained with the patient supine. The image quality however is always compromised. The referrer must always consider the patient's clinical condition and the feasibility of a CXR.

• **Patient location and travel details:** The need for a clinical escort should be conveyed and the points of departure and return and contact details must also be notified to the Imaging Department to ensure the patient is transferred safely and efficiently.

• **Indications:** The CXR can potentially reveal a wide range of pathology and often guides patient management. The referral indications must include salient information regarding the history of the presenting complaint, past medical and surgical history, physical examination findings, results of other investigations and previous imaging. The referral indication should also include a specific question to be answered by the CXR.

• **Contraindications:** It is important to note that the CXR exposes the patient to ionising radiation and the referrer must therefore always consider the clinical need and the significance to management.

Approach to CXR interpretation

When approaching any radiographic image it is essential to have a structured approach. This ensures that all aspects of the image are assessed and that the acquired information is combined with the clinical scenario to proceed to a logical diagnosis. The approach to the CXR includes the following steps:

1 Identify the image and when it was taken
PA erect or semi-erect, AP, mobile AP semi-erect or supine, or lateral.

2 Identify the patient
Full name, sex, age and date of birth.

3 Technical adequacy
• *Orientation* – confirm the right and left markers are correct (usually an 'R' marker is placed on the image indicating the right side).
• *Degree of inspiration/inflation* – the highest point of the right hemidiaphragm should lie between the fifth and seventh anterior

ribs. Hyperinflation may suggest COPD whereas hypoinflation may suggest incomplete inspiration, e.g. due to pain.

• *Field* – are all the areas included in the image (entire chest, first ribs superiorly, humeral heads laterally, and costophrenic angles inferiorly)?

• *Penetration* – the vertebral body outlines should just be visible behind the heart. Their prominence increases in an over-penetrated image but conspicuity of soft tissue lesions decreases. If they are not seen, the image is usually under-penetrated and the lungs will artificially appear whiter. Other causes for not seeing the vertebral bodies include pathological processes such as pleural or pericardial effusions, or physiological causes such as obesity.

The five principal densities seen on plain imaging (see Chapter 1) should be used as references to identify anatomical and pathological structures. These densities should be used to identify the anatomy on the CXR, e.g. airways and lungs, mediastinum, heart, soft tissues, bones and foreign bodies. It is important to remember that adjacent structures of different densities form defined edges. Loss of these edges, or silhouettes, therefore suggests an anomaly and is called the 'silhouette sign'.

4 Artefacts and foreign bodies

Any artefacts or foreign bodies seen on CXR may help target the diagnosis. They may be classified into:

• *External artefacts*, e.g. clothing, oxygen tubing/mask, ECG electrodes and defibrillator pads.

• *Surgical artefacts*, e.g. endotracheal and nasogastric tubes, chest drain, central venous line, prosthetic heart valve, pacemaker/ implantable cardiac defibrillator and wires, arterial stent, sutures/ clips and sternotomy wires.

• *Foreign bodies*, e.g. aspirated radio-opaque objects in the oesophagus or stomach.

Identify normal anatomy and assess pathology

5 Trachea

The trachea descends centrally but is deviated to the right at the level of the aortic knuckle. The trachea may be pulled towards the site of pathology, e.g. lung/lobar collapse and fibrosis, or pushed away, e.g. tension pneumothorax and large pleural effusion.

6 Lungs and pleura

The lungs should have symmetrical radiodensity and be carefully inspected:

• *Lung margins* – absence of lung markings (e.g. pneumothorax), pleural thickening (e.g. mesothelioma, adenocarcinoma and post-inflammatory changes), and calcific deposits (e.g. asbestos exposure).

• *Lung volumes* – loss of lung volume (e.g. pulmonary fibrosis, collapse and pneumonectomy) may be identified by a tracheal and mediastinal shift towards the affected side, narrowing of the ipsilateral intercostal spaces and deviation of the horizontal fissure.

• *Opacities* – opacities should be described in terms of their site, size and imaging characteristics. They may be classified into unilateral or bilateral, and focal or diffuse. Focal and unilateral opacities include inflammatory (e.g. infection) and neoplastic processes. Bilateral and diffuse opacities include pulmonary oedema, atypical pneumonias and structural parenchymal diseases (e.g. pulmonary fibrosis).

7 Mediastinum

The mediastinum may be pulled towards pathology (e.g. collapse and pneumonectomy), pushed away (e.g. tension pneumothorax and pleural effusion), or widened (e.g. lymphadenopathy and aortic aneurysm).

8 Heart

The normal heart measures less than 50% maximum internal width of the thorax on a PA image. This is called the cardiothoracic ratio. Due to cardiac magnification on AP imaging, cardiac dimensions can only be reliably interpreted from a PA image. The cardiac contours should be traced to detect any areas of abnormality (see Chapter 9).

9 Hila

Either hilum can be displaced, enlarged or abnormally shaped. Loss of the normal concave appearance may be the first sign of pathology. If there is an abnormality, assess whether it is unilateral (e.g. bronchogenic carcinoma) or bilateral (e.g. lymphoma and sarcoidosis).

10 Hemidiaphragms

Either hemidiaphragm can be abnormally raised (e.g. volume loss, phrenic nerve palsy, hepatomegaly and diaphragmatic injury). Free gas may be seen beneath the hemidiaphragms (pneumoperitoneum).

11 Review areas

The following areas are important to individually check before completing the CXR interpretation:

• *Costophrenic angles* – fluid (e.g. pleural effusion and haemothorax).

• *Lung apices* – absence of lung markings (e.g. pneumothorax), mass (e.g. Pancoast's tumour) and fibrosis (e.g. TB).

• *Behind the heart* – air-fluid level (e.g. hiatus hernia) and mass.

• *Behind the hemidiaphragms* – fluid (e.g. pleural effusion and haemothorax) and mass.

• *Bones* – ribs, vertebrae, scapulae, clavicles, humerus (e.g. fractures, metastases, myeloma and osteopaenia).

• *Soft tissues* – breast shadows (e.g. mastectomy and tumour), irregular subcutaneous gas (e.g. surgical emphysema) and lymphadenopathy.

10.1 Normal adult male CXR

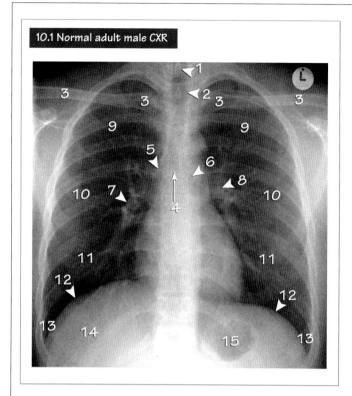

10.2 Normal adult female CXR

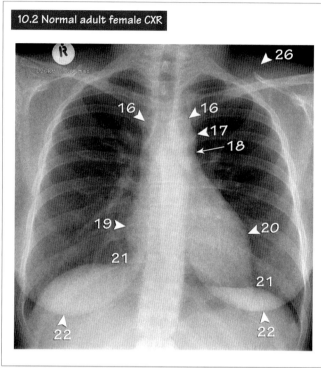

10.3 Normal adult female CXR

Key

1	Spinous process	14	Liver
2	Trachea	15	Stomach bubble
3	Clavicle	16	Sternum
4	Carina	17	Aortic knuckle
5	Right main bronchus	18	Aorto-pulmonary window
6	Left main bronchus	19	Right atrial edge
7	Right pulmonary artery	20	Left ventricular edge
8	Left pulmonary artery	21	Cardiophrenic angles
9	Upper lung zone	22	Breast
10	Middle lung zone	23	Spine
11	Lower lung zone	24	5th rib (left)
12	Diaphragm	25	Scapula
13	Costophrenic angle	26	Fat in soft tissue

Chest anatomy seen on PA CXR

The five principal densities seen on plain imaging (see Chapter 1) should be used as reference points to identify anatomical and pathological structures. It is important to remember that adjacent structures of different densities form defined edges.

Important anatomical landmarks and structures on the normal CXR

Airways and lungs

These are dark areas due to their high air content.

• *Trachea* – seen as a central vertical lucent tubular structure overlying the vertebral column. The right edge of the trachea, otherwise known as the right paratracheal stripe, is usually thin and well defined because it lies adjacent to the air-dense lung. The left edge however lies adjacent to the oesophagus (posterior to trachea) and great vessels (left of trachea) and therefore blends in due to their soft tissue density.

• *Carina* – the bifurcation of the trachea.

• *Right main bronchus* – shorter, wider and more vertical than the left main bronchus. This increases the chance of aspiration affecting the right lung.

• *Left main bronchus* – more horizontal due to its passage over the left atrium of the heart.

• *Left lung* – the upper, lingula and lower lobes are not clearly demarcated on a PA CXR. It is therefore best to describe the location of a lesion in terms of upper, middle and lower lung 'zones'. Each zone can then be compared with its counterpart in the contralateral lung.

• *Right lung* – the upper and middle lobes are delineated by the horizontal fissure, which is often visible. The lower lobe cannot be clearly demarcated from the other lobes. Displacement of the horizontal fissure may help determine the location of a disease process.

Mediastinum

The mediastinum is the middle part of the chest and includes all the organs *except the lungs*, i.e. heart, great vessels, trachea, oesophagus, thymus, lymph nodes, phrenic and vagus nerves. Due to the similar soft tissue densities of these adjacent structures it may be difficult to clearly identify individual structures. The contours of the heart, aorta and trachea are, however, usually identifiable.

Heart

The heart appears as a large soft tissue density structure. The heart borders are made up of the following:

• *Left border* (superior to inferior): aortic knuckle/arch, aorto-pulmonary window, left atrial appendage, left ventricle.

• *Right border* (superior to inferior): SVC, right atrium.

• *Inferior border* (in contact with diaphragm): right ventricle.

Hila

The hila are seen as concave structures formed by the configuration of the divergent pulmonary vessels and bronchi. The *left hilum is usually slightly higher* than the right.

Hemidiaphragms

The highest point of the *right hemidiaphragm is slightly higher* than that of the left to accommodate the liver. A dark rounded area is usually seen under the left hemidiaphragm, which is the *gastric air bubble*. This should not be confused with free intra-abdominal gas, which forms a dark crescent under the diaphragm (pneumoperitoneum).

Costophrenic and cardiophrenic angles

Each hemidiaphragm forms a sharp angle at the point of contact with the thoracic wall, known as the costophrenic angle. Loss or blunting of this angle may be due to lung pathology or fluid accumulation in the pleural space (pleural effusion). Each hemidiaphragm also forms an angle at the point of contact with the pericardium, known as the cardiophrenic angle.

Bones and soft tissues

The bones visible on CXR include:

• *Spine* – lower cervical spine to upper lumbar spine.

• *Sternum.*

• *Ribs.*

• *Clavicles.*

• *Scapulae.*

• *Upper left and right humerus.*

The soft tissues visible on CXR include:

• *Breasts* – may mimic lung shadowing, particularly if large or asymmetric.

• *Normal soft tissues of the neck and thoracic wall* – may be separated by layers of well-defined fat tissue, which appear darker.

11.1 Lobar consolidation

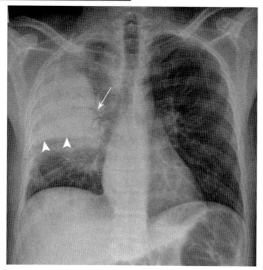

An 'air bronchogram' (arrow) can be seen clearly within the area of shadowing in the right middle zone. This shadowing has a distinct inferior margin (arrowheads) running along the line of the horizontal fissure which is the inferior boundary of the right upper lobe. This is therefore right upper lobe consolidation

11.2 Atelectasis

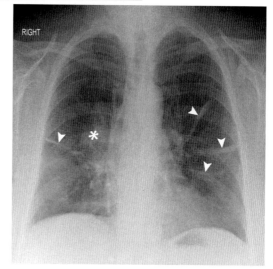

This patient was recovering from a widespread pneumonia when this CXR was taken. There are multiple bands of atelectasis (arrowheads) which are the result of the inflammatory process. There is a persistent area of consolidation in the region of the right hilum (*)

11.3 Bronchiectasis

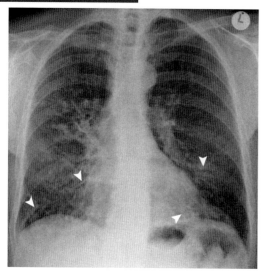

Bronchiectasis is a difficult diagnosis to make with any great certainty on plain CXR imaging. The diagnosis is made accurately on high resolution CT (see Chapter 33). This CXR demonstrates 'tram tracks' (arrowheads) which represent thick-walled dilated bronchi

11.4 COPD

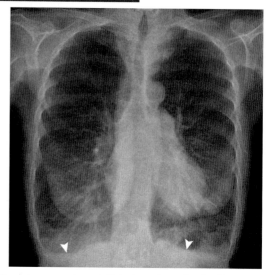

These lungs are hyperinflated as shown by the flattening of the hemidiaphragms (arrowheads). The anterior portion of more than seven ribs can be seen lying above the hemidiaphragms in the midclavicular line on both sides. The lungs are so hyperinflated that the inferior border of the heart is lifted away from the diaphragm

Consolidation

Consolidation is a pathological process caused by filling of the alveolar airspaces with fluid or debris such as:
- *Inflammatory exudates*, e.g. pneumonia (see Chapter 33).
- *Haemorrhage*, e.g. trauma, vasculitis, or pulmonary embolism.
- *Transudates* from various causes, e.g. cardiogenic, nephrogenic, neurogenic, ARDS and drug reactions.
- *Secretions*, e.g. alveolar proteinosis and mucus.
- *Malignancy*, e.g. bronchioalveolar cell carcinoma and lymphoma.

Consolidation appears as a 'fluffy' light grey density that is not well demarcated unless bound by a pleural margin, e.g. a fissure or lung edge. The classic signs are *air bronchograms*, which are dark air-filled branches of the bronchial tree superimposed on a light grey background of fluid or debris-filled alveoli. Other features include loss of the interfaces between consolidated lung and adjacent light grey soft tissue structures, e.g. the left heart border with lingular consolidation, the right heart border with middle lobe consolidation, and the left or right hemidiaphragm with left lower or right lower lobe consolidation respectively. It is important to be vigilant for other associated pathologies, e.g. a pleural effusion, an abscess, or a mass.

Atelectasis

Atelectasis is the incomplete expansion of lung tissue affecting a section or whole of one lung. It is usually not life threatening as normal lung can compensate for the functional loss and the atelectatic area often re-expands once the cause is treated. The causes can be divided into:
- *Obstructive* – a foreign body, tumour or mucous plug may obstruct a large or small bronchus, leading to lobar or lung collapse.
- *Non-obstructive* – a reduction in surfactant production may be the cause of atelectasis in ventilated patients or in ARDS. Surfactant reduces alveolar surface tension and helps splint the alveoli open. Postoperative diaphragm dysfunction is a common cause of atelectasis of the lung bases. Other non-obstructive causes include lung fibrosis and loss of contact between the parietal and visceral pleura, e.g. effusion or pneumothorax, compromising lung expansion.

The CXR appearances depend upon the volume of lung affected. Atelectasis is seen as a focal light grey density and is often linear, especially when located at the lung bases postoperatively.

Bronchiectasis (see Chapter 33)

The CXR can appear normal or non-specific in mild or moderate bronchiectasis. HRCT is the most sensitive imaging modality for evaluating this condition. CXR does however help identify serious disease and therefore remains the first-line investigation for suspicious symptoms such as persistent cough, profuse purulent sputum and recurrent infection. The suggestive CXR features include:
- **Ring opacities** – end-on bronchi with thickened walls appear as circular light grey densities, with black centres, resembling 'rings'.
- **Tram tracks** – side-on dilated bronchi with thickened walls appear as light grey parallel lines.
- **Cystic spaces** – these occur in cystic bronchiectasis and appear as circular light grey densities looking like thin-walled ring opacities. They can be as large as 2 cm in diameter and may contain air-fluid levels.
- **Tubular opacities** – side-on dilated mucus-filled bronchi appear as solid thick light grey densities but are less commonly seen.
- **Crowding of pulmonary vascular markings** – mucous obstruction of peripheral bronchi can cause atelectasis. The loss in lung volume brings the vascular markings closer together.

COPD (see Chapter 33)

The CXR features of COPD include:
- **Lung hyperinflation** – hyperinflation is the most dependable indicator in patients with a history of smoking. The hemidiaphragms are flat and depressed so that *seven or more ribs are visible anteriorly* and a distance less than 1.5 cm exists between the mid-hemidiaphragm and a line connecting the costophrenic and cardiophrenic angles. On a lateral CXR the retrosternal space may be more than 2.5 cm and the AP diameter increases, giving the impression of a 'barrel chest'.
- **Narrow and elongated heart** – hyperinflation may cause the heart to appear narrow, elongated and lifted off the diaphragm. If there is coexisting cardiac failure the heart may appear normal in size or enlarged.
- **Bullae** – parenchymal destruction leads to large black lung areas bordered by light grey hairline densities distorting the surrounding vasculature.
- **Pulmonary vascular pruning** – destruction of lung parenchyma leads to distorted vasculature and reduced lung markings. The central pulmonary arteries and right heart may also be enlarged secondary to pulmonary arterial hypertension.

Lung/pulmonary fibrosis (see Chapter 33)

Pulmonary fibrosis has distinctive features on CXR:
- **Reduced lung volumes** – pulmonary fibrosis is a chronic and progressive condition causing lung scarring, shrinkage and loss of elasticity.
- **Mediastinal shift** – volume loss causes the mediastinum to be pulled towards the fibrosis if unilateral.
- **Reticular/reticulonodular shadowing** – the fibrotic tissue appears as either a light grey meshwork pattern (reticular) or with additional light grey nodular densities (reticulonodular). The distribution of shadowing in the lung varies with aetiology, e.g. ankylosing spondylitis in the upper zone and scleroderma in the lower zone.
- **Ground glass appearance** – in the early stages, a thin 'veil-like' light grey shadow covers all or part of the lung.
- **Honeycombing** – in the advanced stages, a framework of multiple light grey ring-like structures may be seen resembling a honeycomb.
- **Blurring of mediastinum and diaphragms** – fibrotic tissue reduces contrast between the lung and its adjacent soft tissue structures.

Classic CXR features I

• **Consolidation**	'Fluffy' density, air bronchograms
• **Atelectasis**	Focal light grey density and volume loss
• **Bronchiectasis**	Ring opacities, tram tracks, cystic spaces, vascular crowding
• **COPD**	Hyperinflation, elongated heart, bullae, vascular pruning
• **Lung fibrosis**	Volume loss, mediastinal shift, reticulo/nodular shadowing, ground glass, honeycombing

12.1 Cardiomegaly

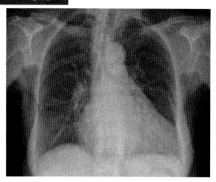

The heart is abnormally large. It takes up greater than 50% of the internal width of the thorax. The patient was known to have left ventricular failure

12.2 Pulmonary oedema

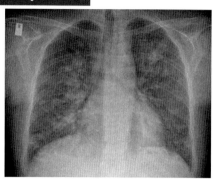

The heart is not enlarged but there are signs of pulmonary oedema with shadowing spreading from the hila. The patient was diabetic and presented with acute myocardial infarction and left ventricular failure

12.3 Kerley B lines

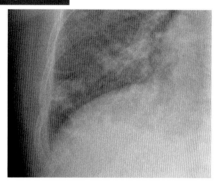

Close-up of costophrenic angle of fig 12.2. Here septal 'Kerley B' lines are seen. These are horizontal lines that reach the pleural surface. They are caused by fluid between the interlobular septa and are a specific sign of pulmonary oedema

12.4 Pleural effusions

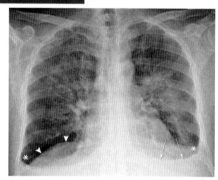

This patient with heart failure has pulmonary oedema and fluid is filling the pleural cavities forming pleural effusions (arrows). The costophrenic angles (*) are blunted. The dome of the diaphragm is still visible (arrowheads)

12.5 Prosthetic heart valves

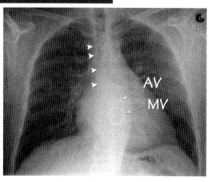

The heart is enlarged due to left ventricular failure. There is evidence of previous cardiac surgery with midline sternotomy wires (arrowheads) and metallic replacements of both the aortic valve (AV) and the mitral valve (MV)

12.6 Asbestos plaques

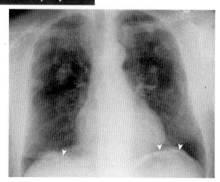

There are multiple dense irregular-shaped opacities over both lungs. These are typical appearances of asbestos plaques. The give-away sign is the layering of dense material over the diaphragm (arrowheads)

Cardiomegaly

Cardiomegaly is an abnormal enlargement of the heart where the *maximum width of the heart shadow is greater than 50% of the maximum internal width of the thorax*. The causes include:

• *Hypertrophy* – caused by an increase in afterload of a particular chamber (e.g. aortic stenosis, hypertension).

• *Dilatation* – secondary to toxic, metabolic, or infectious agents causing myocardial damage.

Hypertrophy of either ventricle does not usually enlarge the heart shadow unless there is synchronous dilatation. Cardiomegaly is usually abnormal, except in athletes, and is associated with other cardiovascular pathology. The shape of an enlarged heart on CXR will depend upon the chamber affected and it may point to the cause:

• A 'globular' shape occurs with pericardial effusion or generalised cardiomyopathy.

• Left ventricular dilatation causes lengthening and rounding of the left heart border and a downward extension of the apex.

• Right ventricular dilatation lifts the apex off the hemidiaphragm.

• Left atrial enlargement causes a double density along the right heart border, comprising the left and right atrial edges. Other signs include left atrial appendage prominence and bronchial splaying of the bronchi at the carina.

Pulmonary oedema

Pulmonary oedema occurs when fluid leaks into the lung interstitium from the pulmonary vasculature, leading to impairment of gaseous exchange. It is caused by either an *increase in vascular hydrostatic pressure* (e.g. cardiogenic causes – left ventricular dysfunction, mitral stenosis), a *decrease in plasma oncotic pressure* (e.g. liver failure, renal failure), or an *increase in pulmonary capillary membrane permeability* (e.g. adult respiratory distress syndrome, aspiration, inhalation injury, neurogenic pulmonary oedema, multiple blood transfusions). The CXR features of pulmonary oedema include:

• **Absence/presence of cardiomegaly** – cardiomegaly is often seen with cardiogenic causes although it may be normal in size in the early stages. The heart is usually normal in size with non-cardiogenic causes.

• **Upper lobe blood diversion** – the upper lobe blood vessels are normally narrower than the lower lobe vessels. In cardiogenic pulmonary oedema, lower zone alveolar hypoxia causes arteriolar vasoconstriction, diverting blood to the upper lobes to optimise gaseous exchange.

• **Alveolar shadowing** – this represents oedema in the alveoli. It predominates in the lower zones if the cause is cardiogenic, and more diffusely if non-cardiogenic. In acute cardiogenic cases, alveolar shadowing spreads out from the hila in the shape of bat's wings.

• **Kerley lines** – these represent interstitial oedema. They are thin linear shadows caused by interstitial fluid or cellular infiltration.

• **Kerley A lines** – these represent distension of channels between peripheral and central lung lymphatics. They are unbranching lines (over 2cm long) extending from the periphery towards the hilum.

• **Kerley B/septal lines** – these represent oedema of the interlobular septa and are characteristic of pulmonary oedema. They are 1 cm long, thin, horizontal and parallel and seen peripherally above the costophrenic angles.

• **Pleural effusions** – pleural fluid causes blunting of the costophrenic angles.

Pleural effusion

Pleural effusion is excess fluid in the pleural space. Aspiration allows biochemical division into transudates (<30g/L of protein) and exudates (>30g/L of protein). Transudates are caused by left ventricular failure, pulmonary embolism and cirrhosis. Exudates are causes by infection, neoplasia and inflammatory conditions, e.g. rheumatoid arthritis or systemic lupus erythematosus. CXR is the primary diagnostic tool for detecting pleural effusions and may point to the cause, e.g. an enlarged heart shadow, lung mass, parenchymal disease, apical fibrosis or bone metastases. Effusions collect in gravity-dependent areas (lung bases when positioned upright). The CXR appearances of pleural effusions include:

• Small effusions *blunt the costophrenic angles with a meniscus*.

• Large effusions can cause *complete 'white-out'* of the lungs, lung collapse and push the mediastinum away from the side of the effusion.

Prosthetic heart valves

Normal heart valves may become dysfunctional due to acute and chronic disease, e.g. bacterial endocarditis, aortic stenosis or rheumatic fever. Replacement valves are designed to restore normal function and may be mechanical or biological tissue grafts. *Mechanical valves are radio-opaque*, appearing as white artefacts within the heart shadow on CXR. The major classes of mechanical valves include 'caged ball', 'tilting disk' and 'bi-leaflet'. A prosthetic mitral valve is larger and aligned more anteroposteriorly than a prosthetic aortic valve, which is smaller and aligned more obliquely on a PA CXR.

Pleural plaques

Pleural plaques are focal areas of pleural fibrosis caused by *previous exposure to asbestos*. Pleural calcification is a late sign, occurring in approximately half of those with asbestos-related disease. It is most easily seen along the diaphragmatic pleura. The CXR features include:

• *Widespread distribution* – commonly mid-lung, paravertebral, diaphragmatic, peripheral and bilateral.

• *Peripheral pleural thickening* – appears as a thickened white line, often non-uniform around the edge of the lung.

• *Calcified plaques* – mimic the appearance of a 'holly leaf' with dense irregular rolled edges and relatively lucent centres.

Plaques evolve slowly and previous CXRs should be reviewed for comparison.

Classic CXR features II

• **Cardiomegaly**	Heart shadow greater than 50% of thoracic cage width
• **Pulmonary oedema**	
(cardiogenic)	Bilateral alveolar shadowing, bat's wings, upper lobe blood diversion, Kerley A lines, Kerley B lines, cardiomegaly, effusion, cardiac pathology signs (sternotomy wires, prosthetic valve, pacemaker/defibrillator)
(non-cardiogenic)	Normal heart size, diffuse alveolar shadowing
• **Pleural effusion**	Costophrenic angle blunting, meniscus, 'white-out'
• **Pleural plaques**	Peripheral pleural thickening, pleural calcific deposits

13.1 Simple pneumothorax

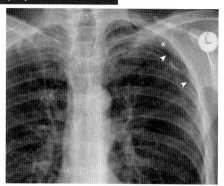

The edge of the left lung can be seen as a thin well-defined line (arrowheads). Beyond this line there are no further lung markings because air is collecting in the pleural cavity (*)

13.2 Chest drain

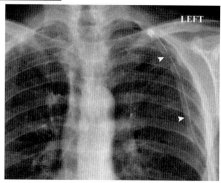

(Same patient as fig 13.1)
A tube has been inserted to drain air from the pleural cavity. It has been placed appropriately with its tip pointing high up towards the apex of the hemithorax

13.3 Tension pneumothorax

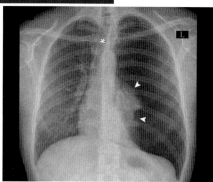

The left lung (arrowheads) is being compressed, the left hemidiaphragm is depressed, and the trachea (*) is pushed towards the right. Immediate aspiration is required

13.4 Hydropneumothorax

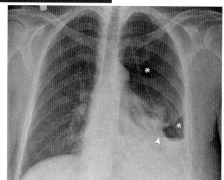

This patient has both a pneumothorax (*) and a pleural effusion (arrowhead) due to an oesophageal rupture. The fluid level does not have the curved meniscus sign of a simple effusion. Note the presence of a chest drain. Haemopneumothorax has identical appearances and is often associated with rib fractures

13.5 Lower left lobe collapse

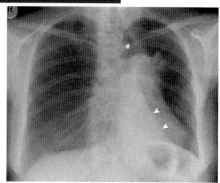

The left lower lobe bronchus is occluded with collapse of this lobe. The edge of the collapsed lobe forms the 'sail sign' (arrowheads). The trachea (*) is pulled towards the side of volume loss

13.6 Right upper lobe collapse

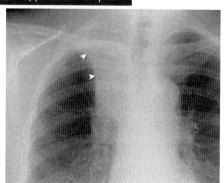

The horizontal fissure (arrowheads) has been pulled upwards due to volume loss of the right upper lobe. The patients in both figs 13.5 and 13.6 had an occluding bronchial carcinoma

Pneumothorax

Pneumothorax is the presence of air in the pleural cavity. During normal ventilation, the thoracic volume increases to create relative negative intrathoracic pressure for lung inflation. However, in the presence of a pleural defect, air enters the potential pleural space and breaks this pressure potential, thereby compromising lung inflation. This impairs gaseous exchange and may cause breathlessness.

• *Simple pneumothorax* is common and occurs in healthy chests, especially in tall, slim, young males. Secondary pneumothoraces can arise in individuals with underlying disease, e.g. COPD, asthma, barotrauma, penetrating chest trauma and pneumonia.

• *Tension pneumothorax* is a medical emergency where air accumulates under pressure in the pleural space due to the formation of a one-way valve at the point of injury, permitting air to enter but not to escape. It can develop from a simple pneumothorax, often following traumatic injury, and requires emergency decompression.

CXR features include:

• *Linear pleural shadow with absence of lung markings beyond* this linear shadow in the peripheral thorax.

• *Air in the pleural cavity will rise to the apices* in an upright CXR. It is therefore vital to review the apical areas.

Haemothorax

A haemothorax is a pleural effusion due to the accumulation of blood within the pleural cavity. It most commonly arises from blunt or penetrating chest trauma. Non-traumatic haemothorax is less common and can result from malignancy, blood dyscrasias, pulmonary infarction and tuberculosis. CXR is the primary diagnostic investigation and the typical appearances on *upright* imaging are *identical to a pleural effusion* (meniscus, blunting of the costophrenic angle, 'white-out' and/or mediastinal shift with a large haemothorax).

Approximately 200–300 mLs of blood is required to obliterate the costophrenic angle on an upright CXR. In the acute trauma setting, however, a portable supine CXR is often the first and only view available upon which management decisions are based. Unfortunately, the presence and size of haemothoraces is extremely difficult to evaluate on supine images. In blunt trauma cases, there may be other associated injuries, e.g. rib fractures, pneumothorax, or damage to the great vessels. These should be excluded on the CXR.

In the context of a traumatic pneumothorax, the presence of a pleural effusion is almost always due to the accumulation of blood in the pleural cavity (haemopneumothorax). There is no meniscal sign due to a direct interface between the pleural air and blood.

Lobar collapse

Collapse of a single lobe causes characteristic patterns on CXR:

• **Right upper lobe (RUL) collapse** – the horizontal fissure is pulled up and there is a soft tissue shadow in the right upper zone. The remainder of the lung expands to fill the void.

• **(Right) middle lobe (ML) collapse** (there is no left middle lobe) – the horizontal and oblique fissures are pulled closer and there is loss of interface between the right heart border and the lung (*silhouette sign*). The lateral CXR demonstrates a wedge-shaped opacity stretching from the hilum anteroinferiorly.

• **Right lower lobe (RLL) collapse** – there is a soft tissue shadow in the right lower zone and loss of interface between the right hemidiaphragm and lung (*silhouette sign*). The collapsed lobe appears as a triangular opacity behind the right heart border without obscuring it. The lateral CXR demonstrates increased density over the lower thoracic spine caused by the shadow of the collapsed lobe.

• **Left upper lobe (LUL) collapse** – there is a 'veil-like' shadow cast over the entire left lung due to the anteriorly lying collapsed lobe. Interposition of the lower lobe between the collapsed lobe and aortic arch may be seen as a crescent of air, known as the *Luftsichel sign*.

• **Lingula lobe collapse** – there is loss of interface between the left heart border and the lung (*silhouette sign*).

• **Left lower lobe (LLL) collapse** – the collapsed lobe is displaced medially and lies behind the heart. A triangular opacity is seen through the heart shadow with a straight left lateral border (*sail sign*). There is also loss of interface between the medial part of the left hemidiaphragm and lung (*silhouette sign*).

Tubes, lines and prostheses

CXR is the usual method for confirming correct positioning of tubes and lines in the chest. On CXR:

• *The tip of an endotracheal tube should be mid-tracheal, 2–3 cm above its bifurcation* at the level of the fourth to fifth thoracic vertebrae. The tip has a radio-opaque marker to enhance its visibility on CXR. If inserted too far, it may enter a bronchus and inflate only one lung causing contralateral collapse.

• *The tip of a central venous catheter should be in the SVC, just above the right atrium.* If it is inserted too far, it may cause arrhythmias through direct contact with the heart. It may also erode through the SVC or right atrium causing haemorrhage and tamponade.

• *The nasogastric tube should follow the central vertical descent of the oesophagus and continue below the left hemidiaphragm into the stomach.* If incorrectly placed, it may enter the trachea or bronchi, perforate the oesophagus or penetrate into the brain through the ethmoid bone.

• *Chest drain* – this tube passes through the chest wall via an intercostal space and its tip lies in the pleural space.

• *Pacemakers and implantable cardioverter defibrillators (ICD)* – these are usually sited below the lateral left clavicle. Pacing wires connect the pacemaker and/or ICD to the heart muscle. Pacemakers may pace one or more heart chambers. ICDs are used in patients at risk of sudden death from arrhythmia.

Classic CXR features III

• **Haemothorax**	Costophrenic angle blunting, meniscus, 'white-out'
• **Pneumothorax**	Linear pleural shadow with absent lung markings in the periphery beyond
• **Collapse of:**	
RUL	Superiorly displaced horizontal fissure, upper zone shadowing
(R)ML	Right heart silhouette sign, wedge-shaped opacity on lateral CXR
RLL	Right hemidiaphragm silhouette sign, lower zone shadowing, increased lower thoracic spine density on lateral CXR
LUL	'Veil-like' shadow, Luftsichel sign
Lingula	Left heart silhouette sign
LLL	Left hemidiaphragm silhouette sign, 'sail sign'

14.1 Lung cancer

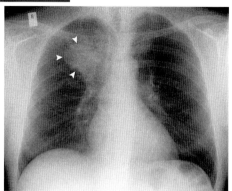

This patient has a large rounded opacity arising from the upper aspect of the right hilum (arrowheads). CT of the chest followed by bronchoscopy and biopsy led to a tissue diagnosis of non-small cell lung cancer

14.2 Metastatic disease

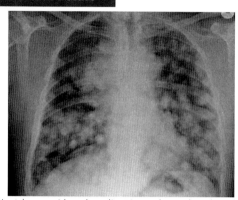

This patient has a widened mediastinum due to lymph node enlargement and numerous small well-defined rounded lung nodules. These are typical features of metastatic disease

14.3 Lung cavity

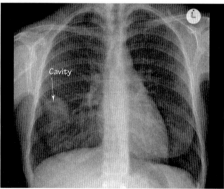

A lung shadow shows a central lucency due to formation of a cavity. This patient had an infected embolus originating from the femoral vein where the patient had injected intravenous drugs

14.4 Bilateral hilar lymphadenopathy

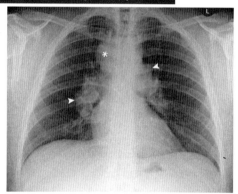

Both hila are enlarged (arrowheads). There is also enlargement of the mediastinum in the region of right paratracheal edge (*). These are classic appearances of sarcoidosis

14.5 Apical scarring due to TB

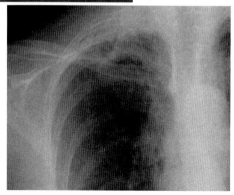

At the lung apex there is irregular fibrotic shadowing. The hilum has been pulled upwards due to volume loss. These features of old TB are often accompanied by calcification

14.6 Thoracic aortic aneurysm

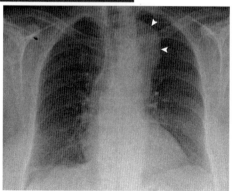

The left side of the aortic arch is enlarged with a smooth contour (arrowheads) due to aneurysmal dilatation of the thoracic aorta

Lung cancer

Approximately 10% of patients with lung cancer are asymptomatic and diagnosed incidentally on CXR. *Primary lung cancer* is the foremost cause of cancer-related mortality in both men and women. Its prevalence is second only to prostate cancer in men and breast cancer in women. The lungs have a rich vascular and lymphatic network, which also predisposes them as a site for *metastatic cancer*. Cancers that frequently metastasise to the lung include thyroid, breast, kidney, prostate, melanoma and bone cancer.

Typical CXR features of lung cancer include:
• *Coin or cavitating lesion* – the centre of the lesion should be closely inspected since some tumours are associated with central cavitation.
• *Multiple* similar-looking lesions suggest metastatic disease.
Indirect CXR features of lung cancer include:
• *Consolidation or collapse* – distal to an obstructing mass.
• *Pleural effusion.*
• *Lymph node enlargement* – mediastinal and/or hilar.
• *Bone metastases.*
• *Malignant lung lesions are rarely calcified* – the presence of calcification suggests an alternative diagnosis e.g. tuberculosis or hamartoma.

It is vital to appreciate that a lung cancer lesion may be hidden by other pathologies or be located behind the heart. Therefore, careful assessment of the retrocardiac area is essential. Comparison with previous CXRs is often helpful in this setting.

Mediastinal lymph node enlargement

Mediastinal nodes drain lymphatics from the lungs, heart, thymus and oesophagus. The causes of mediastinal lymph node enlargement include malignancy (e.g. bronchogenic carcinoma, lymphoma), infection (e.g. tuberculosis, pneumonia, HIV) and inflammatory conditions (e.g. sarcoidosis). Enlarged mediastinal lymph nodes may cause cough, dyspnoea, wheezing, dysphagia, haemoptysis, atelectasis and obstruction of the great vessels, e.g. SVC. There are many lymph node groups within the mediastinum but the hilar nodes are most commonly seen on CXR due to the interface between them and aerated lung. Other mediastinal lymph nodes may be visible on CXR if their enlargement is substantial. It is important to discriminate between nodal enlargement and other soft tissue structures that may produce mediastinal widening, e.g. aortic aneurysm or thyroid goitre.

Tuberculosis (TB)

TB is an airborne mycobacterial infection and most commonly affects the lungs. It can also affect the central nervous system, vascular and lymphatic systems, the urogenital system and bones.

The CXR features of *active* lung TB include:
• *Consolidation* – this can be dense or patchy and may have ill-defined borders.
• *Cavitating lesion* – lucent areas in the upper segments of the lung lobes.
• *Pleural effusion.*
• *Lymph node enlargement* – hilar and/or mediastinal nodes may be enlarged on one or occasionally both sides.
• *Signs of miliary TB* – there may be tiny nodules (1–2 mm) scattered widely throughout the lung parenchyma bilaterally.

The CXR features of *inactive* TB are primarily areas of fibrotic scarring, classically seen in the apex of one or both lungs. This is often accompanied by nodular calcification causing a fibrocalcific appearance. The fibrosis may be extensive enough to cause volume loss resulting in upward displacement of the hilum on the ipsilateral side.

Coin and cavitating lesions

A discrete, approximately circular, area of whiteness seen within a lung field is termed a coin lesion. If the edge is spiculated, irregular or lobulated it is more suggestive of a *malignant lesion*. If the centre of the lesion is more lucent than the edge, this suggests a cavitating process. The differential diagnosis for such lesions is diverse and includes: malignancy (e.g. squamous cell carcinoma), infection (e.g. *Streptococcus pneumoniae, Staphylococcus aureus,* TB, *Klebsiella*) and other rarer causes (e.g. Wegener's granulomatosis, hydatid cyst, rheumatoid nodule).

Thoracic aortic aneurysm

An aneurysm is a localised or diffuse dilation of an artery due to an underlying weakness in the vessel wall. The CXR features of a thoracic aortic aneurysm include:
• *Greater convexity of the right or left superior mediastinum* – this is caused by the soft tissue density shadow of the thoracic aortic aneurysm.
• *Aortic calcification* – atherosclerosis frequently accompanies aneurysm formation and thus calcification is often seen outlining the borders of the aneurysm's soft tissue shadow.

Classic CXR features IV

• **Lung cancer**	Coin lesions or cavitating lesions, single or multiple, usually not associated with calcification, enlarged lymph nodes, consolidation, collapse, pleural effusion, bone metastases
• **Lymph node enlargement**	Lobulated soft tissue masses in the hila and/or mediastinum
• **Tuberculosis** *(common)*	Apical fibrotic and calcific scarring, volume loss, enlarged lymph nodes
(less common)	Pleural effusion, miliary shadowing
• **Thoracic aortic aneurysm**	Widened mediastinum

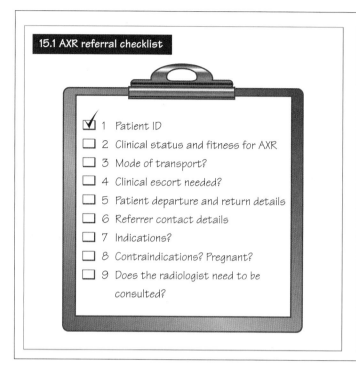

15.1 AXR referral checklist

1 Patient ID ✓
2 Clinical status and fitness for AXR
3 Mode of transport?
4 Clinical escort needed?
5 Patient departure and return details
6 Referrer contact details
7 Indications?
8 Contraindications? Pregnant?
9 Does the radiologist need to be consulted?

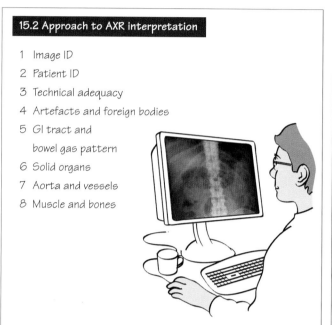

15.2 Approach to AXR interpretation

1 Image ID
2 Patient ID
3 Technical adequacy
4 Artefacts and foreign bodies
5 GI tract and bowel gas pattern
6 Solid organs
7 Aorta and vessels
8 Muscle and bones

AXR referral checklist (see Chapter 7)

The imaging referral form is a legal document. The referrer carries the responsibility to ensure the correct and complete information is conveyed to the Imaging Department so that the patient is appropriately diagnosed and managed.

• **Patient identification:** The referrer must ensure that the Imaging Department receives the correct identification details of the patient to be investigated: full name, date of birth and hospital identification number are the essentials.

• **Clinical status:** The referrer must convey the patient's clinical condition and urgency of the referral to the Imaging Department. In nearly all cases, the AXR is a non-urgent investigation and is superseded by primary resuscitation, and if indicated, other imaging modalities, e.g. CT. If there is doubt a senior team member should consult the radiologist.

• **Patient mobility:** Most AXRs are performed AP supine, thus patient mobility is less of a problem compared with performing a PA CXR. An erect CXR and lateral decubitus films may be requested to assess air-fluid levels and pneumoperitoneum in bowel obstruction, ileus and acute abdominal trauma. In such cases, the referrer must consider the status of the patient and the feasibility of performing such a study.

• **Patient location and travel details:** The need for a clinical escort should be conveyed and the points of departure and return and contact details must also be notified to the Imaging Department to ensure the patient is transferred safely and efficiently.

• **Indications:** The AXR adds a more limited input to the diagnostic process compared with the CXR. However the radiation exposure during an AXR is 35 times higher compared with the CXR. The AXR is most useful in the setting of the acute abdomen, especially in diagnosing bowel obstruction, and may guide further imaging.

• **Contraindications:** It is important to note that the AXR exposes the female reproductive organs to ionising radiation and thus the referrer must take a history of the last menstrual period to check she is not pregnant before requesting an AXR. If there is any doubt and the situation is not an emergency, the referrer should delay the investigation, consider ultrasound, or consult the radiologist.

Approach to AXR interpretation

When approaching any radiographic image it is essential to have a structured approach. This ensures that all the aspects of the image are assessed in a comprehensive manner and the acquired information can then be integrated into the clinical scenario to proceed to a logical diagnosis. The approach to the AXR includes the following steps:

1 Identify the image and when it was taken
AP supine or lateral decubitus.

2 Identify the patient
Full name, sex, age and date of birth.

3 Technical adequacy

• *Orientation* – confirm the right and left markers are correct (usually an 'R' marker is placed on the image indicating the right side).

• *Field* – both hemidiaphragms and hip joints should be visible in the image. In obese patients, the detector cassettes may be used in landscape orientation to include the fuller abdomen.

- *Penetration* – the outlines of the bones of the vertebral column should be visible. If they are not clearly seen the image is under-penetrated. The rest of the image should not be excessively dark, i.e. over-penetrated.

The five principal densities seen on plain imaging (see Chapter 1) should be used to identify anatomical and pathological structures on the AXR, e.g. the hollow gas-filled bowel, soft tissue structures including the solid visceral organs, and the bones. It is important to remember that adjacent structures of different densities form defined edges. Loss of these edges therefore suggests a pathological process and is called the 'silhouette sign'.

4 Artefacts and foreign bodies

The abdomen is a common site for operative intervention and artefacts are common. Furthermore, there are numerous orifices through which foreign bodies may gain access into the body and appear on AXR. Artefacts and foreign bodies may be classified into:

- *External artefacts*, e.g. clothing, nursing objects.
- *Surgical artefacts*, e.g. nasogastric tube, sutures/clips, staples, drains, stomas, suprapubic catheter, vascular stents, gastrointestinal and urological stents, IVC filters and embolisation coils or balloons, and spinal and hip joint prostheses.
- *Foreign bodies* via the oral/nasal route (e.g. hair or foodball bezoars, other radio-opaque objects), the rectal route (e.g. diverse range of radio-opaque objects), the urethral route (e.g. catheter) and the vaginal route (e.g. intrauterine contraceptive devices).

Proceed to identify normal anatomy and assess pathology

5 Gas-filled gastrointestinal tract

The gastrointestinal tract contains gas. It is important to realise that, when lying supine, fluid will displace posteriorly and gas will rise up anteriorly to lie above it. This is why an AP supine AXR will not demonstrate air-fluid levels and thus a lateral decubitus position with a horizontal X-ray beam or CT is required to demonstrate this. Normal variants and pathology that may be seen include:

- *Stomach* – normal pooling of gastric fluid in the fundus may be seen and often termed a pseudotumour.
- *Small bowel* – distension and perforation.
- *Appendix* – appendicolith.
- *Large bowel* – distension, collapse, volvulus, perforation, hernias, diverticular disease, inflammatory bowel disease and intramural gas, e.g. ischaemic bowel.
- *Rectum* – absence of gas secondary to proximal obstruction.

6 Solid organs

- *Liver* – hepatomegaly, small (cirrhotic) and pneumobilia.
- *Gall bladder* – gallstones (only 10% are radio-opaque) and calcified 'porcelain' gall bladder post-chronic cholecystitis.
- *Spleen* – splenomegaly.
- *Pancreas* – difficult to see unless abnormal, e.g. calcification in chronic pancreatitis.
- *Kidneys* – calculi, enlarged kidneys (e.g. obstruction, cysts or tumour), small or atrophic kidneys (e.g. renal artery stenosis or chronic pyelonephritis), abnormal anatomy (e.g. horseshoe kidneys where the lower renal poles cross the psoas margins medially), and pelvic kidneys (e.g. ectopic or transplanted).
- *Adrenal glands* – difficult to see unless calcified (e.g. haemorrhage, malignancy and TB).
- *Ureters and bladder* – calculi, gas in bladder (e.g. fistula, infection, post instrumentation).
- *Uterus and ovaries* – difficult to see but the source of many abnormal pelvic masses in females (e.g. fibroids which may be calcified, ovarian cysts, tumours, teratomas and abscess).
- *Prostate* – usually not seen unless calcifications are present, which are typically seen in the area of the pubic symphysis.

7 Circulatory system

- *Aorta* – aneurysm (often detected incidentally on AXR. While being a silent lethal condition, it is treatable. The AXR diagnosis of abdominal aortic aneurysm could potentially save the patient's life. It is therefore imperative to carefully assess the aorta for calcification and aneurysm).
- *Splenic artery* – calcification and aneurysm.
- *Iliac vessels* – phleboliths (may mimic ureteric calculi).
- *Femoral vessels* – calcification and aneurysm.

8 Muscle and bone

- *Hemidiaphragms* – rupture and phrenic nerve palsy.
- *Psoas muscle margins* – absence of these margins may reflect serious pathology (e.g. leaking blood from an aortic aneurysm effacing the psoas outline).
- *Lower ribs* – malignant metastatic disease, myeloma, fractures and osteoporosis.
- *Vertebral column* – malignant metastatic disease, myeloma, fractures, degenerative disease and osteoporosis.
- *Pelvis* – malignant metastatic disease, myeloma, Paget's disease, fractures and osteoporosis.
- *Sacro-iliac joints* – may be fused in seronegative spondyloarthopathy.
- *Hip joints* – fractures, degenerative disease and prostheses.

16.1 Soft tissues and bones

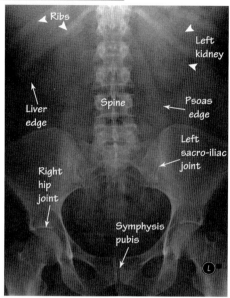

Some soft tissue structures are visible on a normal abdominal X-ray. Here the edges of the liver, kidneys and psoas muscles are clearly seen. Identifiable bones include the ribs, spine, pelvis and femora

16.2 Small bowel

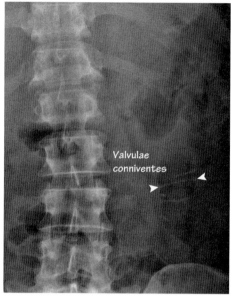

Normal small bowel is often more centrally placed than the colon. It can sometimes be clearly identified by the presence of visible valvulae conniventes (mucosal folds that pass across the whole width of the small bowel)

16.3 Large bowel

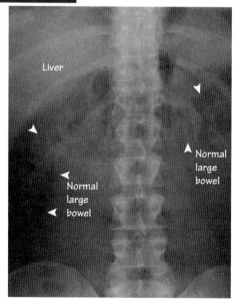

The large bowel (arrowheads) is often seen more peripherally than the central small bowel. The colonic wall is lined by haustra (mucosal folds that do not pass across the full width of the lumen)

16.4 Dense structures

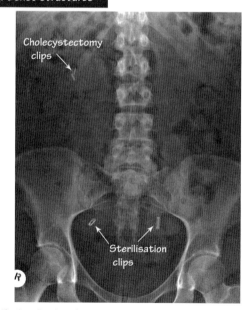

Calcified and other dense structures can often be seen on an abdominal X-ray. This patient has had two previous operations – a sterilisation procedure and a cholecystectomy. Clips left in place for these operations are clearly visible

Abdominal anatomy seen on AXR

The five principal densities seen on plain imaging (see Chapter 1) should be used as reference points to identify anatomical and pathological structures. It is important to remember that adjacent structures of different densities form defined edges.

Important anatomical landmarks and structures on AXR

Gas-filled structures

These are black areas surrounded by grey edges.

• *Stomach* – seen as a subdiaphragmatic ovoid lucency on the left. It should not be confused with free gas which forms a cresentic lucency under the diaphragm.

• *Small bowel* – identified by the following features: central abdominal location, up to 3 cm in diameter, meandering course, presence of transverse valvulae conniventes, usually only contains gas and not stool.

• *Large bowel* – identified by the following features: located peripherally in the abdomen, up to 6 cm in diameter, presence of haustral folds, straight course, usually contains gas and faeces.

• *Rectum* – seen in the presacral area and usually contains gas.

• *Lower borders of lungs* – seen bilaterally below the contour of the diaphragm, as the lung passes behind the dome of each hemidiaphragm into the posterior thoracic recess.

Solid organs

These are indistinct solid grey structures.

• *Inferior border of the heart* – sits on the left hemidiaphragm.

• *Liver* – lies in the right hyopochondrium.

• *Spleen* – lies in the left hypochondrium.

• *Kidneys* – located at the level of T12–L3 with their medial border lying longitudinally parallel to and along the lateral margin of the ipsilateral psoas muscle. The right kidney lies slightly lower than the left due to the position of the liver, and both are three to four vertebral bodies long.

• *Ureters and bladder* – the ureters run distally from the kidney, following a vertical course along the transverse processes of the lumbar vertebrae. The bladder may form a well-defined rounded soft tissue density in the pelvis.

Muscles and bones

The muscles appear as light grey structures and the bones are well-defined white structures.

• *Hemidiaphragms* – left and right.

• *Lateral psoas muscle margins* – run diagonally from the upper lumbar vertebral bodies to the ipsilateral lesser femoral trochanter.

• *Lower ribs* – left and right.

• *Vertebral column.*

• *Pelvis.*

• *Sacrum.*

• *Sacro-iliac joints* – left and right.

• *Hip joints* – left and right.

17.1 Small bowel obstruction

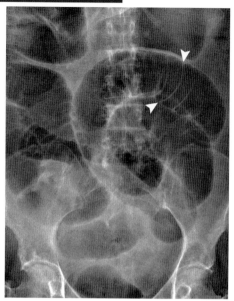

The small bowel is grossly distended. The small bowel is recognised by the visible valvulae conniventes (arrowheads) passing across the width of the lumen. The central position of the loops is another clue

17.2 Sigmoid volvulus

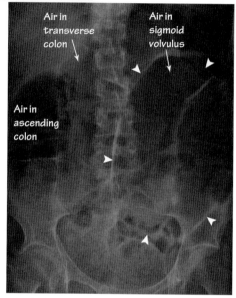

A sigmoid volvulus is seen as a doubled-up loop of bowel in the left iliac fossa forming the 'coffee bean' sign (arrowheads). The volvulus (twist) of the sigmoid colon is causing obstruction of the more proximal colon, which has become distended

17.3 Pneumoperitoneum: Rigler's sign

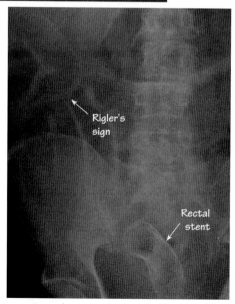

Free intraperitoneal gas can lead to the 'double wall' or 'Rigler's' sign. This is due to the presence of gas/air on both sides of the bowel wall. This patient has a rectal stent in situ which was positioned to bridge an inoperable rectal cancer

17.4 Pneumoperitoneum: Erect CXR

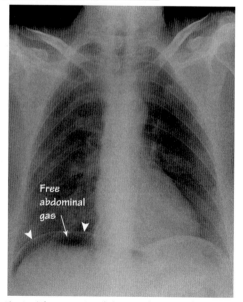

In a patient with an acute abdomen the erect CXR is a far more sensitive investigation than AXR for seeing free intraperitoneal gas. The diaphragm is seen as a thin line (arrowheads) and gas that accumulates underneath it forms a crescent shape

Bowel obstruction

Obstruction of the bowel may be complete or incomplete, acute or chronic, and mechanical or non-mechanical (ileus). The causes include *extramural* (e.g. adhesions, herniae, volvulus and tumour), *intramural* (e.g. Crohn's disease, tumours and strictures), and *intraluminal pathology* (e.g. faecal impaction, gallstone ileus and foreign bodies).

Bowel obstruction can be divided into two types, small and large bowel obstruction, due to the different locations and AXR appearances. The obstructing lesion is often not seen on the AXR but it is important to remember that the bowel proximal to it distends and the bowel distal collapses. The collapsed bowel will therefore not appear on the AXR but identifying this zone of transition will help locate the site of the obstruction. Distal obstructions consequently cause large bowel distension and if there is an incompetent ileocaecal valve, leakage of gas from the large into the small bowel, results in large *and* small bowel distension on the AXR.

Small bowel obstruction (SBO)

The commonest cause of small bowel obstruction is *postoperative adhesions*. Other causes include hernia, Crohn's disease and tumours. The AXR features include:
- The closely spaced folds of small bowel mucosa, known as valvulae conniventes or plica circulares, are seen as *soft tissue densities traversing the entire diameter of the lumen*.
- The *meandering lengthy loops* of small bowel, which are anatomically packaged into the *centre* of the abdomen, are often displaced.
- Luminal contents comprise *gas and fluid*.
- A *diameter greater than 3 cm*, which is the maximum normal diameter for small bowel.

Large bowel obstruction (LBO)

The commonest causes of large bowel obstruction are *tumours* or *strictures*. The AXR features include:
- The widely-spaced haustral folds are seen as *soft tissue densities that classically do not traverse the entire diameter of the lumen*.
- The *straight course* of the ascending and descending colons lies peripherally. The transverse and sigmoid colon lie peripherally or centrally. The rectum lies centrally in the pelvis.
- Luminal contents usually comprise *gas and faeces*.
- A *diameter greater than 6 cm for the large bowel and 9 cm for the caecum*, which are the upper limits of their respective normal diameters.

Volvulus

Torsion of the bowel is known as volvulus. It occurs most commonly in the sigmoid colon or caecum of constipated elderly patients, who have redundant loops of colon on a long mesentery and are therefore at risk of the colon twisting around its mesenteric axis. This is a *surgical emergency* due to the high risk of bowel ischaemia, perforation and death. The AXR features include:
- A grossly *distended inverted U-shaped loop* of sigmoid colon extending from the pelvis to the diaphragm with a curved inner colonic wall.
- RUQ-pointing loop suggests sigmoid volvulus and LUQ- pointing loop suggests caecal volvulus.
- *Loss of the haustral folds* due to distension.
- When two grossly distended loops of bowel are closely apposed, their compressed medial walls form a central cleft, which resembles a *coffee bean* and is therefore called the 'coffee bean sign'.

Bowel perforation

Perforation of the bowel is a life-threatening condition and is therefore a *surgical emergency*. It can occur secondary to iatrogenic procedures and trauma, and many gastrointestinal conditions including peptic/duodenal ulcers, bowel obstruction, volvulus, appendicitis, diverticulitis and toxic megacolon. Patients classically present with an acute abdomen. Bowel perforation is detected by the presence of free gas in the abdomen, i.e. *pneumoperitoneum*. Other causes of pneumoperitoneum should also be considered, e.g. gas-forming peritonitis, rupture of an abscess or the urinary tract, recent abdominal surgery and trauma. It is important to remember that free gas will rise, so the patient's position will determine the location of the gas on the image.

The *supine AXR* features include:
- *Visualisation of the outer and inner surfaces of the bowel walls* due to the presence of gas on both sides. This gives a three-dimensional appearance to the bowel loops and is known as Rigler's sign.
- *Visualisation of the falciform ligament* as a thin, linear, grey line due to the contrasting density between the ligament and free gas (falciform sign).
- A *circular gas lucency* in the central abdomen (football sign).
- Gas *hyperlucency in the right upper quadrant* and prominence of the postero-inferior liver border due to free gas adjacent to the liver.
- *Visualisation of both lateral umbilical ligaments*, which contain the inferior epigastric vessels is called the 'inverted V sign'.

On the *left lateral decubitus horizontal AXR*, the gas rises to between the liver and right hemidiaphragm and is seen as a black pocket density. The *erect CXR* is indicated to detect free gas that rises and collects as *black crescent-shaped lucencies under the hemidiaphragms*. An erect CXR can detect even a few millilitres of gas. It is however important to remember that an erect CXR is not sufficiently sensitive to rule out bowel perforation and a negative erect CXR finding must be interpreted with caution if there is a strong clinical suspicion of bowel perforation. Patients should be put into the correct position 20 minutes before taking the image, to allow sufficient time for the free gas to relocate.

Classic AXR features I

Small bowel obstruction	Meandering, central, contains gas/fluid, distended >3 cm, valvulae conniventes
Large bowel obstruction	Straight, peripheral/central, contains gas/faeces, distended >6 cm (>9 cm caecum), haustral folds
Volvulus	Grossly distended inverted U-shaped colonic loop, loss of haustra, coffee-bean sign
Pneumoperitoneum	
Supine AXR	Football sign, RUQ hyperlucency, falciform sign, Rigler's sign, inverted 'V' sign
Left lateral decubitus AXR	Air between liver and right hemidiaphragm
Erect CXR	Air under hemidiaphragms

18.1 Inflammatory bowel disease

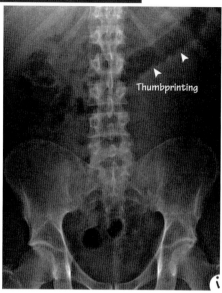

This patient with ulcerative colitis (UC) has an oedematous bowel demonstrated on this AXR as 'thumb-printing' (arrowheads). The descending colon also shows some mucosal thickening but the ascending colon is normal. This is the typical radiographic pattern of UC

18.2 Gallstone and abdominal aortic aneurysm

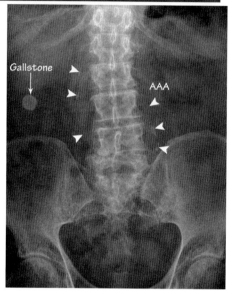

A gallstone is clearly seen in the right upper quadrant. There is also a large abdominal aortic aneurysm (AAA) (arrowheads) seen either side of the lumbar spine. This is visible as it is partly calcified

18.3 Foreign bodies

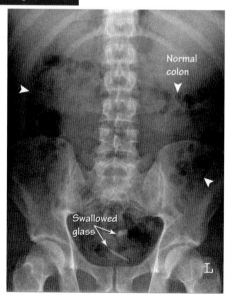

This psychiatric patient swallowed some glass fragments. An AXR was taken to see how far they had travelled and if there was evidence of a complication such as perforation. The glass can be seen clearly over the pelvis. The colonic gas pattern is normal (arrowheads)

18.4 Pneumobilia

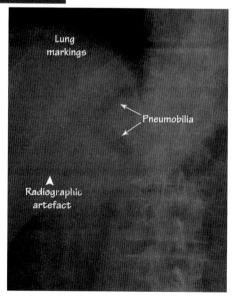

Gas in the biliary tree (pneumobilia) can be seen as branching dark lines in the region of the porta hepatis. This detail of the right upper quadrant shows pneumobilia. Other dark lines, such as the lung markings and artefact seen here, should not be mistaken for biliary gas

Inflammatory bowel disease

Inflammatory bowel disease encompasses a group of chronic inflammatory conditions principally affecting the bowel. The commonest conditions are Crohn's disease and ulcerative colitis and the AXR is primarily used in the assessment of exacerbations and complications. The large bowel normally contains gas and faeces, which solidifies in the descending colon. In inflammatory bowel disease, however, the large bowel may malfunction, causing an absence of solid faecal matter in the descending colon. If the small bowel is involved it may manifest as small bowel obstruction. Crohn's disease and ulcerative colitis are idiopathic but have a range of extraintestinal features, some of which are linked with the HLA-B27 phenotype. These patients may also suffer from sacroiliitis.

Crohn's disease

Crohn's disease is a chronic inflammatory condition *affecting the full thickness of the bowel wall* at any point along the gastrointestinal tract from the mouth to the anus, although most cases involve the terminal ileum leading to malabsorption. It classically occurs in young European adults and has a slight preponderance in females. Crohn's inflammation comprises non-caseating granulomas, which contain Langerhans giant cells. The complications of Crohn's disease include bowel perforation, abscesses and the formation of fistulae and strictures. The AXR features of Crohn's disease include:

• *Discontinuous bowel wall involvement* is seen as 'skip lesions', i.e. regions of affected wall separated by regions of unaffected wall.
• Network of ulceration and wall oedema appears as *cobblestoning*.
• Marked *string-like narrowing of the terminal ileum* due to inflammation or stricture is called the 'string sign'.
• *Small bowel obstruction* secondary to strictures.
• *Air in the urinary tract* secondary to fistula-formation.
• *Sacroiliitis* and *spinal ankylosis*.

Ulcerative colitis

Ulcerative colitis (UC) is a chronic inflammatory condition *affecting the mucosal layer of the large bowel wall*, beginning in the rectum and extending proximally in a continuous fashion. It classically occurs in European adults in their 20s and 30s with a slight preponderance in females. There is also a second peak of patients in their 60s. The inflammation comprises oedematous mucosa, superficial ulceration, crypt abscesses, inflammatory polyps and highly vascular granulation tissue causing bloody diarrhoea. Patients can present with either a distal colitis or a pancolitis. The wall musculature may also be affected, resulting in massive colonic dilatation and is known as toxic megacolon. Furthermore, late in the disease there is increased risk for carcinoma. The AXR features of ulcerative colitis include:

• *Rectal involvement extending proximally and continuous.*
• *Oedematous bowel walls* give the appearance of 'thumbprinting'.
• *Pseudopolyps* appear as areas of thickened mucosa protruding into the lumen.

• Empty large bowel with *rigid featureless walls* lacking haustral folds, giving the appearance of 'lead piping'. This is seen in chronic and so-called 'burnt-out UC' and may be due to muscle spasm or fibrosis.
• *Gross colonic dilatation* or toxic megacolon (also seen in other forms of colitis).

Calculi

A calculus or stone is an abnormal mass comprised of solid material that has precipitated in a bladder or ductal structure. The detection of calculi on plain imaging is dependent on their size and radiodensity.

• **Urinary calculi:** urinary calculi frequently contain calcium and are therefore radio-opaque. Approximately 80% of urinary calculi are seen on AXR, which may be located in the kidney, ureter, or urinary bladder. Occasionally, a large calculus is seen in the renal pelvis with branches into the calyceal system. This is called a *staghorn calculus*. The AXR appearances are usually of a *single, discrete, white, circular opacity in the kidney, ureter, or urinary bladder*.
• **Biliary calculi:** biliary calculi primarily contain cholesterol and are therefore radiolucent and better seen on ultrasound. If however they contain enough calcium, they may be radio-opaque. Approximately 10% of biliary calculi are seen on AXR and are usually located in the gall bladder. The AXR appearances are often of a *collection of multiple, discrete, white, circular opacities, possibly with lucent centres in the gall bladder*.

Foreign body (FB)

There is a vast range of possible FBs that may appear on AXR. The approach to interpretation relies on logical and sometimes imaginative thinking. Initial assessment as to whether the FB is inside or outside the patient's body should be performed. If it is clear that the FB is truly intra-abdominal then the route of entry must be considered (via the mouth, rectum, urethra, vagina, stoma or direct open abdominal wound). While the shape of the FB may be characteristic, it is nevertheless useful to relate its density to the five principal densities on plain imaging (air, fat, soft tissue/fluid, bone and metal) to confirm the diagnosis. Recognition of the AXR appearances of surgical staples, drains and prostheses, as well as anaesthetic tubes and lines, is essential to differentiate between the pathological versus the non-pathological FB. A collection of FB material (often hair or fibre) typically seen located in the stomach is called a *bezoar*.

Pneumobilia

Pneumobilia (gas in the biliary tree) is usually seen after iatrogenic intervention, e.g. ERCP or cholecystoenterostomy. Other causes include sphincter of Oddi incompetence, gallstone ileus, infection, emphysematous cholecystitis, neoplasia or biliary-enteric fistulation. The AXR findings reveal the *outlines of biliary ducts in the right hypochondrium* due to contrasting air within them.

Classic AXR features II

Crohn's disease	Skip lesions, cobblestoning, string sign
Ulcerative colitis	Rectal involvement, proximal and continuous extension, thumbprinting, lead piping, toxic megacolon
Urinary calculus	Single, discrete, white, circular opacity in the kidney, ureter or urinary bladder
Biliary calculi	Collection of multiple, discrete, white, circular opacities with lucent centres located in the gall bladder
Pneumobilia	Appearance of biliary tract outlined in the right hypochondrium

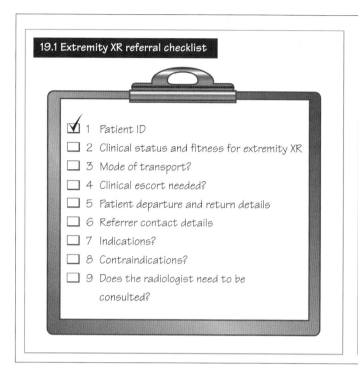

19.1 Extremity XR referral checklist

☑ 1 Patient ID
☐ 2 Clinical status and fitness for extremity XR
☐ 3 Mode of transport?
☐ 4 Clinical escort needed?
☐ 5 Patient departure and return details
☐ 6 Referrer contact details
☐ 7 Indications?
☐ 8 Contraindications?
☐ 9 Does the radiologist need to be consulted?

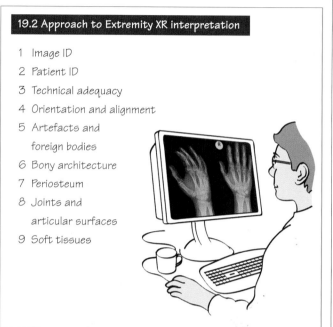

19.2 Approach to Extremity XR interpretation

1 Image ID
2 Patient ID
3 Technical adequacy
4 Orientation and alignment
5 Artefacts and foreign bodies
6 Bony architecture
7 Periosteum
8 Joints and articular surfaces
9 Soft tissues

Extremity XR referral checklist (see Chapter 7)

The imaging referral form is a legal document. The referrer carries the responsibility to ensure the correct and complete information is conveyed to the Imaging Department so that the patient is appropriately diagnosed and managed.

• **Patient identification:** The referrer must ensure that the Imaging Department receives the correct identification details of the patient to be investigated: full name, date of birth and hospital identification number are the essentials.

• **Clinical status and mobility:** Any neurovascular injury of the extremity must be assessed and managed before XR imaging. In trauma cases, the patient should be resuscitated using ATLS guidelines and extremity injuries are therefore usually managed in the secondary survey.

• **Adequate views and extent:** The fundamental difference between plain imaging of the extremity and other body areas is that two views of the site are taken in different planes. The exceptions to this rule include:

1 Rheumatological disease – two views may not be necessary and only indicated regions should be imaged.
2 Hand – AP and oblique views are taken, though a lateral view may be needed for carpometacarpal dislocation.
3 Scaphoid – multiple specific views must be taken to view the scaphoid adequately due to the risk of avascular necrosis with scaphoid fractures.
4 Shoulder – AP and lateral (20° anterior of true lateral) views together with specialised views.
5 Ankle – the AP is not truly absolute and is taken to view the talus within the ankle joint (mortice view).

6 Knee – in trauma cases AP and horizontal beam lateral views are taken to help detect lipohaemarthroses (a fluid level formed by fat floating on blood within the joint).

• **Patient location and travel details:** This needs to be considered carefully depending on patient location. Will the patient return to the referring department? Which mode of transport is the most appropriate and comfortable for the patient? For outpatient referrals consideration must be given to the patient's ability to attend without support.

• **Indications:** There are many indications for extremity XR including fractures and suspected fractures, postoperative progress, rheumatological pain or foreign bodies.

• **Contraindications:** There are few contraindications for XR of the extremity. However, there are definitely contraindications to the positioning needed. These patients may have reduced mobility and this must be considered when requesting specific views.

Approach to extremity XR interpretation

There are various anatomical and technical types of extremity XR and an identical approach may not apply to all. There are however some universal skills that can be applied when approaching any extremity XR, which are logical and systematic so nothing is missed.

1 Identify the image and when it was taken
Anatomical area and orientation of views e.g. AP, lateral, scaphoid or DP (dorsal to plantar – used for plain imaging of the foot).

2 Identify the patient
Full name, sex, age and date of birth.

3 Technical adequacy
• *Orientation* – confirm the right and left markers are correct and whether the radiographer has flagged an abnormality. Ensure the

image is the right way up and has not been digitally flipped. Then assess whether the bones are overlapping and, if so, could this be improved by re-imaging?

• *Fields* – adequate coverage of the bones and joints should be achieved. The series should include images in two planes of the region of interest, together with the joint above and below if imaging a long bone.

• *Penetration* – the bone cortex should be seen within the soft tissue and the soft tissue should be clearly lighter and demarcated from the surrounding air. The five principal densities seen on plain imaging (see Chapter 1) should be used as references to identify anatomical and pathological structures.

4 Artefact and foreign bodies

Jewellery should be removed before imaging but vascular access cannulae or orthopaedic metalwork for fracture or joint repair is often seen on the extremity XR.

The extremities are common sites for foreign bodies, especially glass. Since the visibility of an object depends on its size and relative radiodensity to its surrounding structures, small foreign bodies may be very difficult to see. A surface marker placed at the suspected site before the XR can be useful to help hunt the foreign body on the image.

5 Bony architecture

This must be a meticulous exercise as there are many overlapping lines, which can be misleading. The best technique is to *follow the cortical outlines of each individual bone* and assess the continuity, thickness and definition of the cortex together with the density and architecture of the medulla. If an abnormality is detected within a bone it should be defined in terms of its size, position, width of zone of transition ('narrow' or 'wide' transitional area between normal and abnormal bone), contents (chondroid, osteoid, fat or fluid) and cortical involvement (scalloping, destroyed, expanded).

Assessment of fractures on extremity XR should include:

1 *Location* – which bone and part (e.g. shaft, metaphysis).

2 *Closed* or *open/compound* – skin breached.

3 *Severity* – incomplete (e.g. greenstick or buckle), complete (two pieces), or comminuted (more than two pieces).

4 *Direction* – transverse, oblique, or spiral.

5 *Displacement* – length, translation, angulation, or rotation.

6 *Articular involvement?*

7 *Any underlying bony defect?*

8 *Eponyms* – certain fractures have eponymous names, e.g. Colles' fracture (distal radius fracture with dorsal angulation and displacement) and Bennett's fracture (intra-articular fracture of the first metacarpal base). These names should only be used once the fracture has been described.

9 *Classification systems* – certain fracture types have been systematically classified with respect to the above modalities, e.g. Garden's classification of femoral neck fractures (see Chapter 24) and Weber's classification of ankle fractures (see Chapter 25).

Fracture assessment on extremity XR

1 Location
2 Closed or open (often only detected clinically)
3 Severity
4 Direction
5 Displacement
6 Articular involvement?
7 Any underlying bony defect?
8 Eponyms
9 Classification systems

---

6 Periostium

There are several types of periosteal reaction:

• *Starburst* – due to rapid continuous growth.

• *Lamellated/layered* – due to bursts of quick growth.

• *Stripping* – due to fractures or trauma.

• *Continuous* or *interrupted*.

Starburst and lamellated reaction may be associated with more aggressive bone lesions such as infection or tumours.

7 Orientation and alignment

Are the bones and joints in the correct anatomical alignment? If not, is this acquired or congenital? The convention is to define orientation and alignment by describing the distal fragment in terms of *rotation*, *displacement* and *angulation*.

8 Joints and articular surfaces

A good knowledge of normal joint anatomy is required to evaluate the joints. The following should be assessed:

• Is this the normal anatomical joint alignment?

• Is the joint subluxed or dislocated?

• Is there a defect of the articular surface?

• Is there new bone growth or a subchondral defect?

9 Soft tissues

The soft tissues often hold clues to the nature of the pathology and careful inspection is time well spent to glean this information. Displacement of muscles by fluid or enlarged fat pads may be seen (e.g. haematomas, joint effusions and soft tissue masses). The soft tissue should also be carefully examined to detect any irregular subcutaneous gas, which could represent *surgical emphysema* or may be due to a *gas-producing infective organism*.

20.1 Normal shoulder: AP view

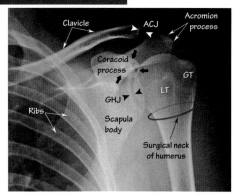

This is a standard view for looking at the shoulder joint. The bones, joints, lung and soft tissues are visible. The surgical neck of the humerus is a common site of proximal humeral fracture. The GHJ is perfectly aligned. GHJ glenohumeral joint, ACJ acromioclavicular joint, GT greater tubercle, LT lesser tubercle (of humerus)

20.2 Normal shoulder: Y-view

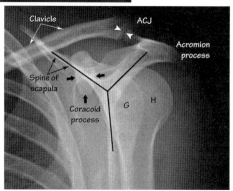

On this view the scapula forms a Y shape comprising the body, spine and acromion process. The humerus (H) overlies the glenoid (G) and lies behind the coracoid process. ACJ acromioclavicular joint

20.3 Normal shoulder: axial view

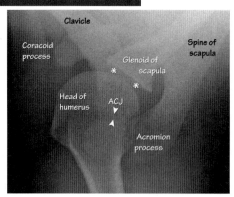

This view is taken with the patient's arm abducted, but is often not tolerated by the patient if there is restriction of movement due to pain. The view gives a clear indication of glenohumeral joint (*) alignment. The head of the humerus is seen to lie behind the coracoid process

20.4 Normal elbow – 13-year-old boy: lateral and AP views

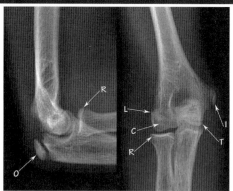

The ossification centres of the elbow are demonstrated. These form the mnemonic 'CRITOL' according to the order of their appearance. C capitulum, R radial head, I internal (medial) epicondyle, T trochlea, O olecranon, L lateral epicondyle

20.5 Normal hand: oblique and AP view

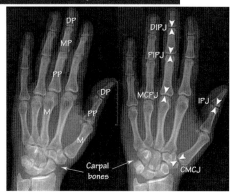

M metacarpal bone, PP proximal phalanx, MP middle phalanx, DP distal phalanx, CMCJ carpometacarpal joint, IPJ interphalangeal joint (thumb only), MCPJ metacarpophalangeal joint, PIPJ proximal interphalangeal joint, DIPJ distal interphalangeal joint

20.6 Normal wrist/carpal bones: AP with ulnar angulation

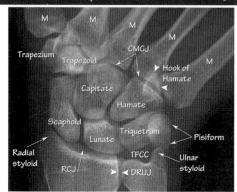

In this view the wrist is stressed towards the ulnar side in order to 'open' any fracture present in the scaphoid. CMCJ carpometacarpal joint, RCJ radiocarpal joint, DRUJ distal radio-ulnar joint, TFCC position of triangulofibrocartilage complex, M metacarpal bone

Upper limb anatomy seen on XR

Plain X-ray imaging demonstrates the normal bony anatomy of the limbs very well, however, normal soft tissue structures are less well seen. The important bony landmarks are centred around the joints. The anatomical position is used for description (standing with palms forwards). The five principal densities seen on plain imaging (see Chapter 1) should be used as reference to identify anatomical and pathological structures.

Shoulder

AP and 'Y' views are commonest. The shoulder bones include the proximal humerus, scapula, lateral end of clavicle and upper ribs.
• *Proximal humerus* – this has a 'head', which sits in the glenoid of the scapula and forms the synovial ball-and-socket glenohumeral joint. The 'anatomical neck' forms an insertion surface of the glenohumeral joint capsule. The surgical neck is a common site for fractures. The greater and lesser tubercles form attachment points for the rotator cuff muscles (subscapularis, supraspinatus, infraspinatus, teres minor).
• *Scapula* – this has a glenoid fossa, which articulates with the humeral head and has attachment points for the long head of biceps and the long head of triceps muscles. The acromion is the highest point of the shoulder and articulates with the lateral end of the clavicle, forming the synovial acromioclavicular joint. The coracoid process is a curved structure, which projects anteriorly from the scapula and lies just below the lateral end of the clavicle. This is an attachment point for the pectoralis minor, coracobrachiali, and short head of biceps muscles.
• *Clavicle* – this is a curved bone connecting the scapula to the sternum. It provides stability for the arm to be raised above the head and has attachment points for the trapezius, deltoid and pectoralis major muscles.
In the 'Y' view, the head of the humerus is seen positioned over the glenoid fossa with the coracoid process projecting anteriorly from the scapula.

Elbow

AP and lateral views are the most common. The elbow bones include the distal humerus and the proximal radius and ulna.
• *Distal humerus* – this is comprised of the medial and lateral epicondyles, capitulum which articulates with the radius, trochlea which articulates with the ulna, and the olecranon fossa which lies posteriorly to accommodate the olecranon of the ulna and contains the posterior fat pad. The posterior fat pad is not normally visualised on a lateral view and if seen indicates a joint effusion, which in the context of trauma is highly suggestive of an intra-articular fracture even if the bones appear normal. Anteriorly, the coronoid fossa accommodates the coracoid process of the proximal ulna and contains the anterior fat pad. The anterior fat pad can be a normal variant on a lateral view, unlike the posterior fat pad.
• *Proximal radius* – this is cylindrical and lies lateral to the wider and bulkier proximal ulna. It has a 'head' which articulates with the capitulum of the humerus proximally and the radial notch of the ulna medially, 'neck', and radial tuberosity which is an attachment point of the biceps muscle.
• *Proximal ulna* – this is broad and lies medial to the narrow proximal radius. It comprises the olecranon which projects superiorly and sits in the olecranon fossa of the humerus and articulates as a hinge joint with the trochlea of the humerus, radial notch which articulates with the radial head and permits pronation of the radius over the ulna, and

ulnar tuberosity which is an attachment point for the brachialis muscle. In children, the bony landmarks of the elbow are only identifiable once they have ossified. The time order of these ossification centres is crucial to identify normal anatomy from pathology.

Elbow ossification centres

The ossification centres ossify in the following order:

C	Capitulum of humerus (1 year)
R	Radial head (5 years)
I	Internal/medial epicondyle of humerus (7 years)
T	Trochlea of humerus (9 years)
O	Olecranon of ulna (10 years)
L	Lateral epicondyle of humerus (11 years)

Wrist

AP and lateral views are the most common. The wrist bones include the distal radius and ulna, eight carpal bones, and proximal metacarpals.
• *Distal radius* – this is broad and lies lateral to the narrow distal ulna. The distal radius has a bifaceted surface to articulate with the scaphoid and lunate in the proximal carpal row. This articular surface is angled laterally and towards the palm to form the radial styloid. The distal radius also has an articulation with the distal ulna to form the distal radioulnar joint (DRUJ).
• *Distal ulna* – this is narrow and lies medial to the broad distal radius. It does not articulate directly with the proximal carpal row but does articulate with the radius at the DRUJ and forms attachment for the clinically important triangulofibrocartilage complex (TFCC) which lies between the ulnar styloid and the triquetrum.
• *Carpal bones* – the eight carpal bones are divided into two rows:

Carpal bones (lateral to medial)

Proximal row	Scaphoid, lunate, triquetrum, pisiform
Distal row	Trapezium, trapezoid, capitate, hamate

Hand

AP and oblique views are the commonest. The hand bones include the metacarpals, phalanges and sesamoids.
• *Metacarpals* – these are numbered lateral to medial and each has a 'base' proximally, a 'shaft', and 'head' distally. The base of the first metacarpal articulates with the trapezium, the second with the trapezoid, the third with the capitate, the fourth with both the capitate and hamate, and the fifth with the hamate. The metacarpal heads articulate with their respective proximal phalanx at a metacarpophalangeal joint (MCPJ).
• *Phalanges* – these are numbered lateral to medial. The thumb only has proximal and distal phalanges, which articulate through an interphalangeal joint. The remaining four digits have proximal, middle and distal phalanges that articulate through a proximal and distal interphalangeal joint (PIPJ and DIPJ).
• *Sesamoid bones* – there are commonly sesamoid bones associated with the anterior surface of the thumb at the metacarpophalangeal joints.

Extremity XR anatomy II: pelvis and lower limb

21.1 Normal pelvis and hips: AP view

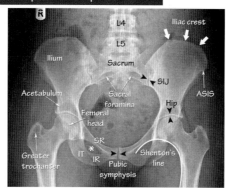

SIJ sacroiliac joint, ASIS anterior superior iliac spine, SR superior ramus, IR inferior ramus (of pubis), IT ischial tuberosity, (*) obturator foramen. Shenton's line is formed by the SR and medial border of the femur

21.2 Normal hip: lateral view

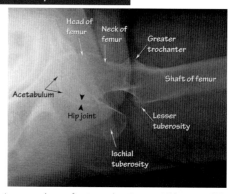

A lateral view may show a fracture that is not visible on an AP view. To achieve this view the contralateral hip is abducted with the knee flexed to avoid overlap of structures. This position is hard to hold, especially for patients in pain, and is often of limited value

21.3 Normal knee – 13-year-old: AP view

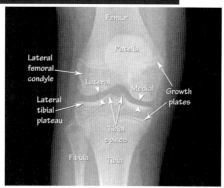

The knee joint consists of three compartments – the lateral, medial and patellofemoral compartments. The lateral and medial joint spaces (arrowheads) are clearly seen on an AP view. The epiphyseal growth plates are unfused in this 13-year-old. These should not be mistaken for a fracture

21.4 Normal knee – 13-year-old: lateral view

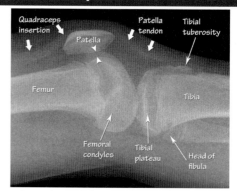

With a lateral view the patellofemoral joint (arrowheads) is visible. The patella is the largest sesamoid (intratendinous) bone in the body. The quadriceps tendon which inserts into the upper aspect of the patella and the patellar tendon which passes from the patella to the tibial tuberosity are clearly seen

21.5 Normal ankle joint: lateral and AP/mortise view

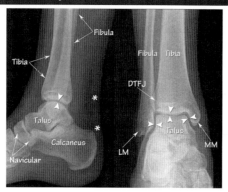

Both these views are centred on the ankle joint (arrowheads). DTFJ distal tibiofibular joint, LM lateral malleolus (distal fibula), MM medial malleolus (distal tibia), (*) soft tissue density of the Achilles tendon

21.6 Normal foot: oblique and dorsoplantar view

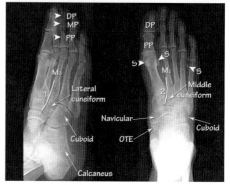

The 3rd metatarsal bone (M3) is aligned with the lateral cuneiform (line 1) and the 2nd metatarsal bone (M2) is aligned with the middle cuneiform (line 2). Sesamoid bones (S) are a common and normal finding. Accessory ossicles are common and although a normal finding may cause symptoms as in this patient who has an os tibiale externum (OTE). PP proximal phalanx, MP middle phalanx, DP distal phalanx

Pelvis and lower limb anatomy seen on XR

Plain X-ray imaging demonstrates the normal bony anatomy of the pelvis and lower limbs, but normal soft tissue structures are less well seen. The five principal densities seen on plain imaging (see Chapter 1) should be used as references to identify anatomical and pathological structures.

Pelvis

AP view is the commonest. The pelvic bones include those of the pelvic ring, femora and lower lumbar vertebrae.
• *Pelvic ring* – the bones include the sacrum, coccyx, ilium, ischium and pubis. There are two sacroiliac joints (SIJs) and a pubic symphysis. The female pelvis is broader than the male with a wider basin.
• *Sacrum* – this lies at the base of the spine and is formed by fusion of five vertebrae. It articulates with the ilium bilaterally at the fibrosynovial SIJ.
• *Coccyx* – this is formed by fusion of four vertebrae and is attached to the inferior tip of the sacrum.
• *Ilium* – the two iliac bones consist of large blades, which form surfaces for attachment for muscles of the back, buttock and leg. It also forms part of the acetabulum. The anterior superior iliac spine (ASIS) is an attachment point for the inguinal ligament and sartorius muscle. The anterior inferior iliac spine (AIIS) is an attachment point for the rectus femoris muscle and iliofemoral ligament.
• *Ischium* – the two ischia comprise the posteroinferior aspects of the pelvic ring bilaterally and include the ischial spine and ischial tuberosity. It also forms part of the acetabulum. The ischial tuberosity forms a surface for attachment of the hamstring muscles and supports body weight when sitting.
• *Pubis* – the two pubic bones are located anteriorly and articulate with each other through the cartilaginous pubic symphysis. Each has a superior and inferior ramus and pubic tubercle, which is an attachment point of the inguinal ligament. The pubis forms part of the acetabulum and also provides attachment surfaces for the adductor muscles.

Hip

AP and lateral views are the commonest. The hip bones include the acetabulum and the proximal femur.
• *Acetabulum* – this is cup-shaped and located in the anterolateral pelvis. It is formed by the coalescence of the ilium, ischium and pubis.
• *Proximal femur* – the 'head' sits in the acetabulum forming the synovial ball-and-socket hip joint. The major blood supply to the head runs distal to proximal within the 'neck', a common fracture site. The greater trochanter (lateral) is an attachment point for the gluteal muscles. The lesser trochanter (medial) is an attachment point for the iliopsoas muscle.
On the lateral view, an imaginary line drawn longitudinally through the middle of the femoral neck normally passes through the head. On the AP view, normal alignment of the femoral neck can be traced by 'Shenton's line' (smooth imaginary line following the inferior edge of the superior pubic ramus and running along the medial edge of the femoral neck and shaft).

Knee

AP and horizontal beam lateral views are the commonest in the context of trauma. The knee bones include the distal femur, patella, proximal tibia and fibula.
• *Distal femur* – this has lateral and medial condyles, which articulate with the tibial plateau. The intercondylar fossa has attachment surfaces for the anterior and posterior cruciate ligaments (ACL and PCL).
• *Patella* – this is the largest sesamoid bone of the body. It overlies the superior aspect of the articular surface of the distal femur and articulates with the femur at the patellofemoral joint.
• *Proximal tibia* – this has a plateau divided into medial and lateral compartments by the anterior and posterior tibial spines, which are attachment points for the cruciate ligaments. The plateaus are lined superiorly by cartilaginous cushions called menisci and articulate with the femoral condyles. The tibial tuberosity lies on the anterior proximal tibial surface and is where the patellar tendon attaches.
• *Proximal fibula* – this is a narrow long bone, lying lateral to the tibia. Its 'head' lies below the level of the tibial plateau and is not part of the knee joint.

Ankle

Mortise and lateral views are the commonest. The ankle bones include the distal tibia, distal fibula and talus.
• *Malleoli* – the medial malleolus comprises the medial edge of the distal tibia. The lateral malleolus comprises the distal fibula. The posterior malleolus comprises the posterior distal tibia.
• *Syndesmosis* – this is the broad ligament of the tibiofibular articulation and is not seen on plain X-ray imaging. Widening of this articulation indicates syndesmotic damage, often related to a fibular fracture.
• *Talus* – the dome of the talus lies within the mortise, formed by the distal tibia and fibula.

Heel

• *Calcaneus* – this articulates with the talus and cuboid and has a trabecular pattern. It is orientated with a 'Bohler's angle' of 20–40° at the intersection between a line drawn from the top of the tuberosity to the top of the posterior facet and a second line drawn from the top of the posterior facet to the top of the posterior process (see Figure 25.5).

Foot

Dorsal to plantar (DP) and oblique views are the commonest. The foot bones include the anterior margin of calcaneus, head of talus, midfoot bones (navicular, cuboid and cuneiforms), metatarsals and phalanges.
• *Metatarsals and cuneiforms* – the lateral edge of the first metatarsal and medial edge of the second metatarsal should be in line with the corresponding edges of the medial and middle cuneiforms respectively. The metatarsal heads articulate with their respective proximal phalanx at a metatarsophalangeal joint (MTPJ).
• *The base of the fifth metatarsal* – peroneus brevis muscle attaches here and is a common site for avulsion fractures.
• *Big toe* – the first metatarsal and phalanges are normally in line. Medial displacement of the first metatarsal with lateral displacement of the phalanx is seen in hallux valgus.

22.1 Anterior shoulder dislocation: AP view

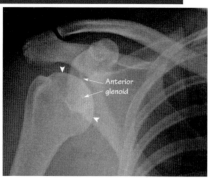

The surface of the humeral head (arrowheads) does not align with the line formed by the anterior rim of the glenoid fossa. There has been no visible bony fracture

22.2 Anterior shoulder dislocation: axial view

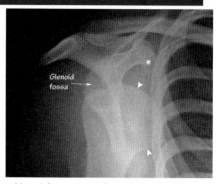

The humeral head (arrowheads) is displaced forwards out from the glenoid fossa and now lies under the corocoid process of the scapula (*). This indicates an anterior dislocation

22.3 Pathological fracture

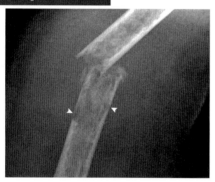

There is a transverse fracture of the mid-shaft of the humerus. There are areas of lucency of the bone trabecular pattern and in places there is loss of cortical thickness (arrowheads). The patient had multiple myeloma

22.4 Clavicle fracture

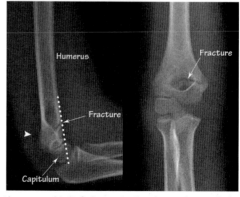

There is a midshaft fracture of the clavicle. The distal part is pulled downwards by the weight of the arm and the proximal part is pulled up by the sternocleidomastoid muscle

22.5 Radial head fracture

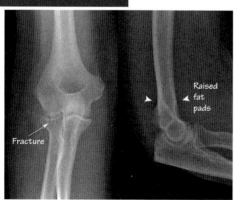

The AP view (left) shows a fracture passing through the radial head into the elbow joint. There are raised fat pads (dark) seen both at the front and back of the distal humerus on the lateral image (right). In the context of trauma it indicates an intra-articular fracture even if no fracture is seen

22.6 Supracondylar fracture

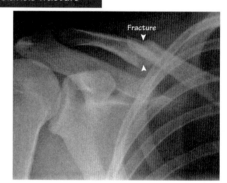

Less than one-third of the capitulum lies in front of the anterior humeral line (dotted), indicating a fracture which is seen clearly on both views. There is a raised posterior fat pad (arrowhead) which is a sign of an accompanying joint effusion

Shoulder dislocation

Anterior

Anterior shoulder dislocations are common and usually related to initial abduction and then extension of the arm, which levers the head anteriorly bringing it to lie inferomedial to the glenoid. This final position gives the characteristic clinical sign of flattening or indentation of the lateral aspect of the deltoid muscle. The injury may be associated with axillary nerve damage and this must be assessed and documented before and after any intervention. Further bony injuries may include fracture of the greater tuberosity, anterior glenoid rim and a 'Hills-Sachs' lesion (depression fracture of the posterolateral aspect of humeral head after impaction with the glenoid). Other soft tissue injuries include brachial plexus, axillary artery and Bankart lesions (anterior tear of glenoid labrum).

The required views include AP and lateral scapular or axial view, although these may be technically challenging due to pain. The humeral head is seen displaced anteromedial to the glenoid.

Posterior

Posterior shoulder dislocations are uncommon and often associated with tonic seizures, especially if bilateral. On plain X-ray, the 'light-bulb' sign is usually identified (humeral head exits glenoid and rotates to give a symmetric light-bulb shape on the AP view).

Classic XR features of shoulder dislocation

Anterior	Humeral head inferomedial to glenoid
Posterior	Light-bulb sign

Pathological fractures

Pathological fractures are often associated with low-impact mechanisms and occur through bone softened by osteoporosis, tumours or cysts. The shafts of long bones and vertebrae are common sites. Initial investigations include plain X-ray imaging of the long bone injury site, which frequently reveals a transverse fracture. The underlying bone must be evaluated carefully for areas of lucency, abnormalities of trabecular pattern, and loss of cortical thickness. If a pathological fracture is suspected, further investigations are then required including biochemical tests (bone disease, systemic disease), tumour markers, skeletal survey and biopsy. Causes of pathological fractures include metastases (breast, lung, thyroid, kidney, prostate cancers), generalised bone disease (metabolic bone disease, osteoporosis, Paget's disease), local bone disease (bone cyst, chronic infection, fibrous cortical defect) and primary bone tumours (osteosarcoma, chondrosarcoma, Ewing's tumour).

Classic XR features of pathological fractures

- Transverse fracture from low-impact injury
- Lucent areas
- Abnormal trabecular pattern
- Loss of cortical thickness

Clavicle fracture

Clavicle fractures are usually caused by a violent fall onto an outstretched hand or a direct blow to the tip of the shoulder. The lateral fragment is pulled inferomedially due to the weight of the arm and the medial end is pulled superiorly by the action of the sternocleidomastoid muscle. In adults the fracture takes three weeks to allow some return of function, however it takes six weeks for complete recovery. The fracture heals with a callous which may be uncomfortable and unsightly. Complications include vascular and lung damage, non and malunion.

Acromioclavicular joint separation

The acromioclavicular joint is a synovial joint, which can be injured by a downward force on the shoulder tip causing tenderness over the joint with some degree of deformity. On plain X-ray imaging, the inferior clavicular border should be aligned with the inferior acromial border.

Radial head fractures

The radial head can be injured by a fall onto an outstretched hand. Radial head fractures are classified into:

- *Undisplaced fractures* – these are often difficult to see on plain X-ray imaging; however, associated features can be used to identify the fracture (e.g. posterior fat pad seen as an area of lucency at the posterior aspect of the distal humerus is abnormal and indicates a joint effusion). If no further fracture is seen and the clinical signs and symptoms are suggestive, then an undisplaced radial head fracture can be assumed. These are usually managed with analgesia and a sling.
- *Displaced fractures* – the radius should align with the capitulum of the humerus. These fractures should be corrected to minimise the risk of developing painful restriction to supination and pronation.
- *Comminuted fractures* – these are managed according to severity (e.g. open reduction and internal fixation or complete excision of the radial head with prosthetic replacement).

Supracondylar fractures

Supracondylar fractures are extra-articular and account for 55% of elbow fractures in 2–14-year-olds. They can occur following a fall onto an outstretched arm causing swelling (and sometimes deformity) and the child is typically unwilling to move it. The immediate complications include brachial artery and median nerve injury and therefore neurovascular status must be assessed before and after any manipulation, as well as on initial examination. If there are signs of ischaemia (pulselessness, pallor, pain, paraesthesiae, paralysis), this must be addressed before imaging. AP and true lateral images are usually required (on the lateral view a line down the anterior cortex of the humerus should normally have a third of the capitulum lying anterior to it). Rotation of the distal humeral fragment and presence of abnormal fat pads must also be evaluated. Management involves closed reduction with a cast or open reduction and internal fixation. Other complications include anterior compartment syndrome (causing compression of median nerve and radial artery), Volkman's ischaemic contracture, malunion (leading to anatomic and functional deformity) and myositis ossificans (post-traumatic calcification of muscle).

Upper limb XR classic cases II: forearm, wrist, and hand

23.1 Colles' fracture: lateral and AP views

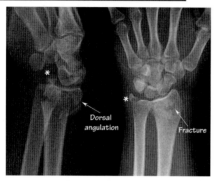

A transverse fracture of the distal radius is clearly seen on both views. Dorsal angulation of the distal component and an accompanying fracture of the ulnar styloid (*) are classic features of a Colles' fracture

23.2 Scaphoid waist fracture: AP view

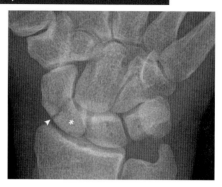

A fracture (arrowhead) passes across the waist of the scaphoid. Failure to treat this injury leads to a high risk of avascular necrosis of the proximal pole (*). This fracture is often not detected on X-ray and so clinical suspicion should lead to treatment with clinical and radiological follow-up

23.3 Monteggia fracture-dislocation: lateral view

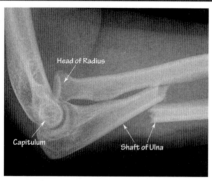

A transverse fracture of the ulna shaft is accompanied by dislocation of the head of radius from the capitulum of the humerus

23.4 Greenstick fracture: AP and lateral views

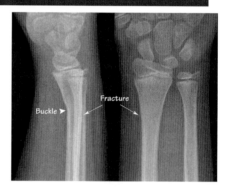

A transverse fracture of the distal radius breaches the dorsal cortex and buckles the ventral cortex. These are typical features of a greenstick fracture

23.5 Boxer's fracture: AP and oblique views

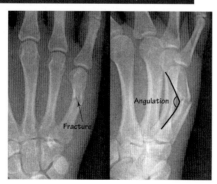

There is a transverse fracture of the little finger metacarpal with palmar angulation of the distal component. This common fracture is said to relate to poor fighting skills. This patient had punched a wall in anger while intoxicated

23.6 Rheumatoid arthritis: both hands

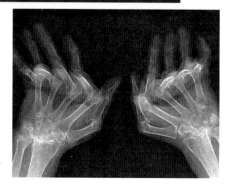

Severe changes of rheumatoid arthritis are shown. These include loss of the carpal joint spaces, erosions of the metacarpal joints and volar subluxation of the metacarpophalangeal joints with ulnar deviation of the phalanges

Distal radius and ulna wrist fractures

• **Colles' fracture** – this is a very common wrist fracture and is usually seen in elderly osteoporotic patients, following a fall onto an outstretched hand. The patient typically attends with a painful wrist, which has a 'dinner fork' deformity and radial deviation of the wrist and hand. The fracture is within 2.5 cm of the wrist joint and has dorsal angulation and displacement of the distal radial fragment. There is frequently an associated fracture of the ulnar styloid. Imaging includes AP and lateral views of the wrist but, if the diagnosis remains unclear, MR imaging may help. If good reduction can be achieved then immobilisation may be adequate management. Complications include damage to the median nerve and extensor pollicis longus which usually require surgical intervention.

Classic XR features of Colles' fracture

• Lucent distal radius fracture line (sclerotic line suggests impaction)
• Shortened radius
• Distal fragment displaced and angulated dorsally (distal radius has a normal volar angulation of 0–22°)
• Ulnar styloid fracture may be present
• No articular involvement (unlike Barton's fracture)

• **Smith's fracture** – this is a distal radius fracture, where the distal fragment is palmar (volar) displaced and usually results from a fall onto the arm with the wrist in flexion. These fractures are unstable and will most often require open reduction and internal fixation.

• **Barton's fracture** – this is a distal radius fracture, which involves the articular surface of the distal radius and therefore predisposes to joint pain, stiffness and osteoarthritis.

Radius and ulna fractures

The intimate association of the radius and ulna at their proximal and distal ends forms a ring. If one part of the ring is broken, there may be a another break elsewhere.

• **Monteggia fracture** – this usually arises from a direct blow to the forearm. This is an ulnar fracture with an associated radial head dislocation at the elbow.

• **Galeazzi fracture** – this usually arises from a fall onto an outstretched hand with a flexed elbow. This is a radial shaft fracture with distal radioulnar subluxation.

• **Greenstick fracture** – this is an incomplete fracture where one side of the cortex has broken and the other side is bent but still in continuity. It commonly occurs in the forearm of children due to the pliability of their bones and derives its name from the similar pattern seen in a broken young tree branch.

Carpal injuries

• **Scaphoid fracture** – this is usually caused by a fall onto a dorsiflexed outstretched hand or violent hyperextension of the wrist. The patient classically presents with swelling at the wrist and pain in the 'anatomical snuffbox'. The blood supply to the scaphoid bone enters the bone distally and travels proximally to supply the proximal pole. Fractures of the scaphoid waist have a high risk of disrupting the blood supply, which can cause avascular necrosis (AVN) of the proximal fragment if not treated. It is often difficult to appreciate scaphoid fractures on plain X-ray imaging and therefore, if there is clinical suspicion, multiple views are taken. If the clinical suspicion is high but a fracture is not identified, it cannot be excluded and the patient should be managed empirically with repeat clinical and radiological assessment in 10–14 days. If diagnosis remains uncertain, MR imaging may provide the answer.

• **Perilunate dislocation** – hyperextension injuries can dislocate the lunate from the carpus leaving it attached to the radius. This injury can be easily missed on AP views but is readily seen on lateral views. The median nerve is at risk of damage with severe disability if left untreated.

• **Trans-scaphoid perilunate dislocation** – this is the combination of perilunate dislocation with an associated scaphoid waist fracture. This fracture pattern is present in 70% of perilunate dislocations. The proximal scaphoid pole remains attached to the lunate.

Osteoarthritis of the hand (see Chapter 24)

Osteoarthritis (OA) of the wrist and hands is due to wear and tear and commonly involves the distal (DIPJ) and proximal interphalangeal joints (PIPJ), trapezoscaphoid joint and first carpometacarpal joint. Patients classically present with joint pain, deformation and crepitus, which is worse after use. Osteophytes are noticeable as lumps around the DIPJs (Heberden's nodes) and PIPJs (Bouchard's nodes).

Classic XR features of hand OA

• Joint space narrowing
• Articular surface sclerosis
• Subchondral cyst formation
• Osteophyte formation
• Radial subluxation of the first metacarpal base

Rheumatoid arthritis of the hand

Rheumatoid arthritis (RA) is a chronic systemic inflammatory disease causing synovial overgrowth (pannus), leading to destruction of cartilage and bone resulting in joint deformation. The deformities include radial deviation of the wrist, ulnar deviation and subluxation of the metacarpophalangeal joints (MCPJ), damage to extensor tendons causing PIPJ hyperextension with DIPJ hyperflexion (swan neck deformity) and PIPJ flexion with DIPJ hyperextension (Boutonniere deformity), and hyperextension of the interphalangeal joint with fixed flexion and subluxation of the MCPJ in the thumb. Patients classically present with morning stiffness and symmetrical painful swelling of the MCPJs, PIPJs, wrist joints, but typically sparing of the DIPJs. The stiffness seems to improve with use.

Classic XR features of hand RA

• Periarticular swelling and osteopenia, loss of fat planes (early changes)
• Joint space narrowing
• Erosions where cartilage has been lost
• Joint subluxation/dislocation, joint fusion (late changes)

Metacarpal fractures

Metacarpal fractures such as the 'boxer's' fracture (usually distal fifth metacarpal fracture caused by a blow with a clenched fist) are commonly seen in the Emergency Department. Patients typically present with a swollen painful hand and may offer a spurious history incongruous to the injury. Rotation, shortening and angulation are repaired if marked and both AP and oblique views of the hand are required to accurately assess the injury. A true lateral view is required if a carpometacarpal dislocation is suspected as it can lead to severe disability if not treated.

24.1 Neck of femur fracture (NOFF): AP view

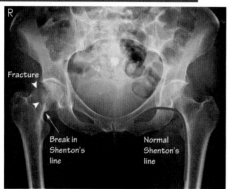

Shenton's line is normal on the left (red line). If this line is followed on the right a clear breach in the cortex is seen along the neck of the femur. A fracture line passes across the femoral neck from this point (arrowheads)

24.2 Osteoarthritis: AP view

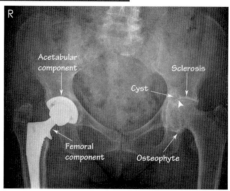

The left hip shows joint space narrowing (arrowhead), articular surface sclerosis, subchondral cyst formation, and an osteophyte of the head-neck junction. The right hip has already been replaced

24.3 Paget's disease: left hip AP view

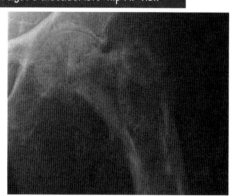

Coarsening of the trabecular markings and thickening of the cortex are typical features of Paget's disease

24.4 Slipped upper femoral epiphysis: 'frog-leg' view

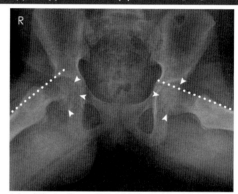

On the right (R) the 'line of Klein' (dotted line) no longer passes through the femoral capital epiphysis (arrowheads). Normal appearances are shown on the left

24.5 Perthes' disease: AP and 'frog-leg' views

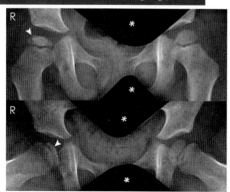

The right femoral epiphysis is small and flattened compared with the left side. Sclerosis of the epiphysis (arrowheads) and joint space widening are also demonstrated. Shielding (*) is used to protect the genitals from radiation exposure

24.6 Developmental dysplasia of the hip (DDH): AP view

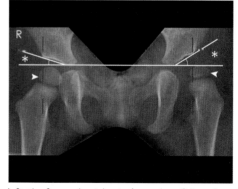

On the left the femoral epiphysis (arrowhead) lies almost entirely outside Perkins' line (red dotted line). The acetabular angle (*) is also increased on the left. Normal appearances are shown on the right

Neck of femur fracture (NOFF)

These are common injuries, often sustained by the elderly. The patient classically presents unable to weight-bear on a shortened and externally rotated leg (due to the unopposed action of the iliopsoas muscle on the femur). NOFFs are clinically classified into:

• *Intracapsular NOFF* – these are high transcervical or subcapital fractures within the joint capsule and disrupt the major blood supply to the femoral head. This predisposes the femoral head to avascular necrosis (AVN) or fracture nonunion. These fractures require hemiarthroplasty or total hip replacement.

• *Extracapsular NOFF* – the fracture lies outside the joint capsule (lower third of the neck) and so the vascular supply to the femoral head is uninterrupted. These can be treated with dynamic hip or cannulated screws, thereby preserving the femoral head.

• *Trochanteric NOFF* – these can be divided into pertrochanteric (through both trochanters), intertrochanteric (between the trochanters) and subtrochanteric. Pertrochanteric and intertrochanteric fractures occur from a twisting motion and usually require internal fixation. Subtrochanteric fractures are often pathological.

Plain X-ray interpretation of NOFF

Two views are required: AP and lateral projections.

• AP view – 'Shenton's line' should be traced (along the inferior edge of the superior pubic ramus, passing on to medial edge of femoral neck and shaft). Discontinuity suggests fracture.

• Lateral view – the femoral neck and head should be in continuity so that a longitudinal line through the middle of the femoral shaft runs through the femoral head.

Intracapsular NOFFs are classified radiologically using the Garden classification.

Garden classification of intracapsular NOFFs

I   Incomplete subcapital fracture with valgus impaction and interruption of trabecular lines across the joint

II Complete but undisplaced fracture with normal trabecular lines across the joint

III Complete and partially displaced fracture with interruption of trabecular lines across the joint

IV Complete and fully displaced fracture with interruption of trabecular lines across the joint

---

Pelvic ring fracture

Stable fractures

Stable fractures are usually single bone injuries (e.g. pubic bone, wing of ilium, avulsion fractures). Pubic rami fractures are more common in osteoporotic patients and are usually uncomplicated, requiring analgesia and physiotherapy. However, some may be complicated by damage to the urethra, bladder or pelvic blood vessels.

Unstable fractures

Complex fractures arise from disruption to the main pelvic ring. These are usually unstable and require orthopaedic management.

• *'Open book' fracture* – anteroposterior compression produces a lateral rotation fracture with disruption of the posterior elements in combination with fractures of the pubic rami or disruption of the pubic symphysis. This can lead to catastrophic haemorrhage from the iliac vessels and requires fixation (i.e. 'closing the book').

• *Hemipelvis rotational fracture* – external compression from a direct blow to the pelvis or hip from the side causes disruption of the posterior and/or anterior elements with the hemipelvis rotated inwards. The treatment depends on the severity (from bed rest to surgery).

• *Anterior and posterior shear fracture* – vertical compression from a fall causes shearing of the posterior and/or anterior elements. Sacral plexus injury can lead to neurological deficit.

Osteoarthritis of the hip

Osteoarthritis (OA) is a degenerative disease with progressive joint surface breakdown. Damage to the cartilage leads to loss of proteoglycans from its matrix and increased water uptake, which causes cartilage thickening. Further erosion leads to proteoglycan and collagen release into the synovium, resulting in chronic synovitis. This eventually leads to remodelling of the joint with mal-loading and compensatory new bone formation, thereby further propagating the disease. OA of the hip usually presents with pain, reduced range of movement and altered function.

Classic plain XR features of hip OA

• Joint space narrowing
• Articular surface sclerosis
• Subchondral cyst formation
• Osteophyte formation (new bone at articular surface edges)

Paget's disease

This is an idiopathic multifocal bone disease characterised by increased resorption and disordered bone formation, commonly affecting the axial skeleton and skull. The bones are prone to fracture as they become thickened and deformed. The incidence increases with age and there may be malignant change.

Paediatric hip lesions

• **Slipped upper femoral epiphysis (SUFE)** – this is a displacement of the upper femoral epiphysis from the femoral neck and commonly affects overweight boys during their *adolescent* growth spurt. It usually has insidious onset of hip pain, limp and shortening and external rotation of the affected leg. On plain X-ray imaging the femoral head is displaced posteromedially with loss of physeal definition, best seen on 'frog-leg' views (supine with feet brought up towards gluteal muscles and knees relaxed laterally). The 'line of Klein' (line drawn along superior edge of femoral neck) on AP view no longer intersects the proximal epiphysis.

• **Perthes' disease** – this is osteonecrosis (avascular necrosis) of the upper femoral epiphysis due to a vascular anomaly. The femoral head becomes soft and reforms over a few of years. It may affect children from *five to ten years of age*. On plain X-ray imaging the affected head is smaller with epiphyseal sclerosis and joint space widening. Later, the reformed head is larger and flatter or may even be fragmented.

• **Developmental dysplasia of the hip (DDH)** – this is a developmental deformity of the acetabulum due to abnormal interaction with the femoral head, leading to severe disability if not treated within the *first months of life*. It is far commoner in females and clinically detected by limited abduction and posterior subluxation (Ortolani/Barlow tests). Ultrasound is used for initial evaluation, but once the femoral heads calcify, plain AP X-ray imaging is performed to assess 'Perkins' line' (vertical line drawn from the lateral rim of the acetabulum) and 'Hilgenreiner's line' (line connecting superolateral aspects of acetabular triradiate cartilage). The calcified femoral head focus should lie inferomedial to the intersection of these lines. An 'acetabular angle' greater than 30° indicates dysplasia (measured between Hilgenreiner's line and slope of the acetabular roof).

Lower limb XR classic cases: knee, ankle and foot

25.1 Tibial plateau fracture: AP knee

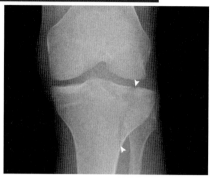

A vertical split fracture is seen on the lateral side of the tibial plateau (arrowheads)

25.2 Tibial plateau fracture: lateral knee

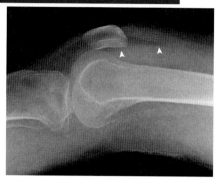

The fracture is not easily seen on this view but a fat-blood interface is seen (arrowheads). This is known as a lipohaemarthrosis (fat and blood in a joint)

25.3 Ankle fracture

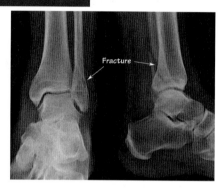

Fracture

There is an oblique fracture of the lateral malleolus (distal fibula). This is at the level of the ankle joint and can therefore be classified as a Weber B type fracture

25.4 Lisfranc injury

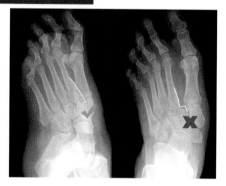

This is an example of how some injuries are only visible on one view. The DP (dorsiplantar) view (right) shows loss of alignment of the medial edges of the second metatarsal and the middle cuneiform. Alignment appears normal on the oblique view (left)

25.5 Calcaneal fracture

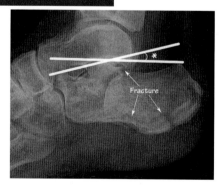

Fracture

There is flattening of the calcaneus with reduction of Bohler's angle (*) to 15° (normally 20-40°). Multiple fractures involving the subtalar joint were caused by falling from height and landing on the heels. The patient also had spinal injuries – a common combination

25.6 Osteoarthritis

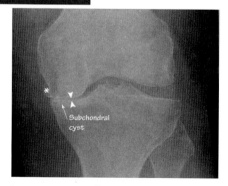

Subchondral cyst

The knee is a common site for osteoarthritis. Here there is loss of the medial joint space (arrowheads) with articular surface sclerosis (increased density of bone) and formation of subchondral cysts. A large marginal osteophyte (*) is also present. These are the four cardinal features of osteoarthritis

Tibial plateau fractures

These fractures are often complex and include vertical split and depression fractures. The full extent of injury is frequently difficult to appreciate on plain X-ray imaging and requires further imaging, for example with CT, before planning surgery. Plain X-ray imaging may demonstrate a lipohaemarthrosis. Fractures of the lateral plateau are the most common, associated with a high impact force, and have the worst prognosis. They are usually caused by impaction of the lateral femoral condyle on the tibial plateau.

Lipohaemarthrosis

Lipohaemarthrosis is fat and blood within a joint. The term is used in radiology to indicate fat/blood fluid level appearances in a joint on plain X-ray imaging. This is caused by *layering of fat and blood*, due to their different densities (fat layer floats on blood layer). Lipohaemarthrosis is most readily seen in the suprapatellar pouch of the knee joint on the horizontal beam lateral view. The fat originates from the bone marrow and its presence indicates the presence of an intra-articular fracture, which may otherwise be subtle.

Osteoarthritis (OA) of the knee (see Chapter 24)

The knee is a common site for primary presentation of OA. One or both of the knee joint compartments may be affected, causing a deformity of the leg. A valgus deformity arises when the leg below the knee is displaced outwards, away from the midline of the body. The reverse is true in a varus deformity.

Classic XR features of knee OA

- Joint space narrowing
- Articular surface sclerosis
- Subchondral cyst formation
- Osteophyte formation (new bone at articular surface edges)

Ankle fractures

Trauma to the ankle can result in injuries to the distal tibiofibular ligaments, syndesmosis, medial ligaments, lateral collateral ligaments and the medial, lateral and posterior malleoli. 85% of sprained ankles involve the lateral collateral ligaments. Different mechanisms produce different patterns of injury. The Weber classification of ankle fractures is derived from the mechanism of injury and describes various fracture patterns.

Weber classification of ankle fractures

A Distal fibular fracture
   Supination injury
   Ligaments intact
B Fibular fracture at level of ankle joint
   Supination/external rotation injury
   Distal tibiofibular ligaments damaged (may require surgery)
C Fibular fracture proximal to ankle joint
   Pronation/external rotation injury
   Ligaments damaged (usually requires surgery)

Calcaneal fractures

The calcaneus is usually injured following a fall from height. Care should be taken to exclude other injuries in the axial skeleton (e.g.

vertebral fractures) as the force is transmitted up the body. These fractures are difficult to fully appreciate on plain X-ray imaging and often require CT imaging. Lateral and axial views are usually required.

Lisfranc fracture

This is a midfoot injury and the name given to a tarsometatarsal fracture dislocation. The injury is sustained by landing on a plantar flexed foot with a rotational component or by a heavy object landing on top of the foot. The metatarsals are displaced laterally (typically second to fifth) but this finding can be easily missed on plain X-ray imaging with potentially severe complications including joint degeneration and compartment syndrome. Careful assessment of the bony alignment is therefore critical. The lateral edge of the first metatarsal and the medial border of the second metatarsal should be aligned with the corresponding borders of the medial and middle cuneiforms respectively. The lateral edge of the fourth metatarsal should align with the lateral border of the cuboid.

Gout of the great toe

This is a crystal arthropathy, most often seen in men over 40 years of age due to the deposition of urate crystals (which are positively bire-fringent on microscopy) in the joint. Dehydration, diuretic use and soft tissue destruction can precipitate an attack. The patient typically presents with a hot, swollen first metatarsophalangeal joint. The plain X-ray imaging features do not usually appear for 6–12 years following the initial attack.

Classic XR features of gout

- Joint effusion with periarticular swelling
- Joint space preservation
- Eccentric erosions with thin sclerotic margins and elevated overhanging margins
- No periarticular osteopaenia
- Proliferative bone changes (bone clubbing)

Calcium pyrophosphate dehydrate (CPPD)

CPPD deposition may be asymptomatic, lead to clinical syndromes similar to gout (pseudogout), or mimic rheumatoid arthritis or osteo-arthritis. CPPD deposition is sometimes associated with metabolic diseases such as hyperparathyroidism or haemochromatosis and gives rise to the classic radiological appearance of chondrocalcinosis (calci-fied cartilage), which is most commonly seen in the wrists or knees. CPPD is often considered synonymous with pseudogout, but in fact it has more X-ray features in common with osteoarthritis, such as joint space narrowing. In CPPD however the distribution is more symmetrical and in this respect it is similar to rheumatoid arthritis.

Stress fractures

These are caused by minor trauma leading to micro-fractures, which are propagated by repeated stress. They commonly occur in the meta-tarsals and tibia of military recruits and sports people. They are often hard to visualise on plain X-ray imaging and only a small periosteal reaction of the related bone may be seen. MRI of the forefoot however is much more sensitive. Micro-fractures usually heal with rest, with callous formation.

26.1 Normal: OM 30° view

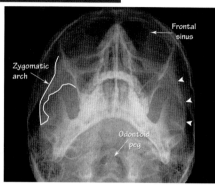

The 'elephant's trunk' of the zygomatic arch (white line and arrowheads) is clearly seen on this view. Note also the frontal air sinuses and the odontoid peg

26.2 Blowout fracture: OM view

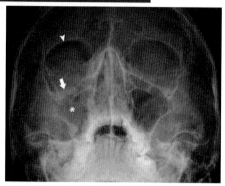

The thin orbital floor (arrow) is depressed with opacification of the maxillary sinus (*) due to blood. Air entering the orbit from the maxillary sinus gives rise to the 'black eyebrow' sign (arrowhead)

26.3 Tripod fracture: OM view

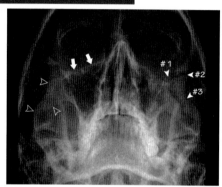

There is a complex fracture involving the orbital floor (#1), lateral orbital wall (#2) and zygomatic arch (#3). Note the normal orbital floor (arrows) and the normal zygomatic arch (open arrowheads) on the right

26.4 Tripod fracture: CT 3D reformat

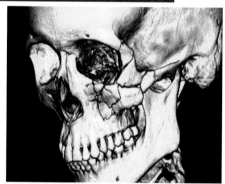

This CT of the same patient as in fig 26.3 reveals a more complex fracture than is appreciated on plain XR. CT can be a useful planning tool before facial surgery

26.5 Mandible fracture: OPG

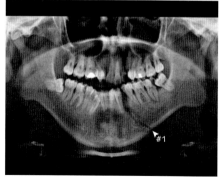

Blunt trauma to this patient's jaw has caused an obvious fracture (#1). A second fracture should be suspected and further views may be required

26.6 Mandible fracture: PA mandible view

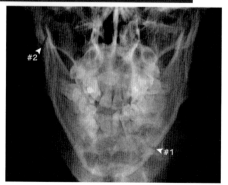

On this view of the same patient as in fig 26.5, the first fracture (#1) is less obvious, however a second fracture (#2) is clearly seen which in hindsight is visible on the OPG

Face anatomy seen on XR

There are several standard plain XR views used to demonstrate the bony anatomy of the face. Structures of the face are anatomically complex, and CT may therefore be required for a more complete assessment of facial fractures or other pathology.

• *Occipitomental view (OM)* – this permits good views of the frontal and maxillary bones, which make up the largest portion of the face. Together with the zygomatic bones they form the bony orbital rim. The zygomatic bone also articulates with the zygomatic process of the temporal bone to form the zygomatic arch, seen as an 'elephant's trunk' on both the OM and OM30° views.

On the OM view the occiput and odontoid peg of the C2 vertebra are projected over the facial bones.

The frontal, ethmoid and the pyramid-shaped maxillary air sinuses are clearly seen on the OM view. The infraorbital foramen passes through each maxillary sinus below each orbit. This contains the infraorbital artery, vein and nerve, and a branch of the maxillary nerve (trigeminal nerve).

The thin orbital roof separates the orbital contents from the anterior cranial fossa. It is made up of the frontal bone and the lesser wing of the sphenoid. The orbital floor separates the orbit from the maxillary sinus and is comprised of the zygomatic bone and maxilla. The apex of the cone-shaped orbit, which forms the optic canal for passage of the optic nerve, is comprised of the greater and lesser wings of the sphenoid. The medial orbital wall is comprised of the ethmoid and lacrimal bones.

• *OM30° view* – the X-ray beam is angled approximately 30° more steeply than the OM view. This allows a second view of the face and provides more accurate assessment of the inferior orbital rims and maxillary sinuses.

• *Orthopantomogram (OPG)* – this view is taken dynamically with the X-ray machine rotating around the patient to provide a panoramic view of the mandible. The mandible's ramus, angle and body are seen clearly without overlapping their contralateral side. The hyoid bone is visualised on both sides of the image. Other structures seen include the coronoid process, which acts as an insertion site for the temporalis muscle, and the condylar processes, which articulate with the temporal bone to form the temporomandibular joints. The mandibular canal, which transmits the inferior alveolar nerve, artery and vein is seen passing through the ramus and body of the mandible.

• *PA mandible view* – the mandible forms a bony ring, and as with any rigid ring, a fracture almost always comprises two breaks, or one break with an associated dislocation. If there is a visible fracture and doubt exists about the site of a second fracture, a specific view of the mandible can be performed.

• *Foreign body (FB) views* – specific views are performed for assessment of FBs depending on the position of the injury. For location of intraocular FBs, two views may be taken with the eyes looking upwards and then downwards.

Approach to facial XR interpretation

In the context of trauma the standard OM and OM30° views should be checked for fractures around the orbital rims, walls of the maxillary sinuses, and on the upper and lower surface of the 'elephant's trunk' of the zygomatic arches. Lines passing across the upper aspect of the fontal sinus, the bridge of the nose and across the alveolar process below the nasal cavity should also be checked for fractures.

The sinuses (especially maxillary and frontal) should be assessed for opacification or an air-fluid level. In the setting of trauma this may represent blood within the sinus, which should raise the suspicion of a nearby fracture. The orbit and cranial vault should be inspected for evidence of air, which may suggest fracture of the ethmoid or frontal sinus, or of the cranial vault.

Blow-out fracture

Blunt eye trauma can lead to increased intraorbital pressure with decompression through a fracture of the thin orbital floor. The inferior rectus muscle may be entrapped, resulting in diplopia. On XR there may be herniation of intraorbital soft tissue through the fracture and opacification of the maxillary sinus by blood. However, the tell-tale appearance is of air entering the orbit, giving rise to the 'eye-brow' sign.

Tripod fracture

This is caused by blunt trauma to the cheek resulting in a comminuted fracture of the zygomaticomaxillary complex involving the orbital floor, the lateral orbital wall and zygomatic arch. The infraorbital nerve may be damaged if the infraorbital foramen is involved, with sensory loss in the affected cheek. As with many facial fractures, CT is often required for accurate analysis.

Le Fort fractures

These are uncommon fractures caused by blunt trauma to the mid-face and first described by French surgeon René Le Fort.

• *Le Fort I* – a horizontal fracture running across the lower maxilla, back to the ptyergoid plates.

• *Le Fort II* – a complex pyramid-shaped fracture that travels from the nasal bridge, inferolaterally through the medial orbital rim, vertically across the maxillary sinuses, and beneath the zygomatic bones to the pterygoid plates.

• *Le Fort III* – this is a transverse fracture of the face with dissociation of the face from the cranium. The fracture travels posteriorly from the nasal bridge along the medial wall of the orbit, and then back along the lateral orbital wall to the maxillofrontal suture and then passes down through the zygomatic arch.

Fractured mandible

Mandibular fractures are usually caused by blunt trauma to the jaw. There are nearly always two or more fractures or dislocations ('ring' phenomenon). The muscles attached to the fracture fragments may displace the proximal segment upward and medially, or conversely may stabilise the bony fragments.

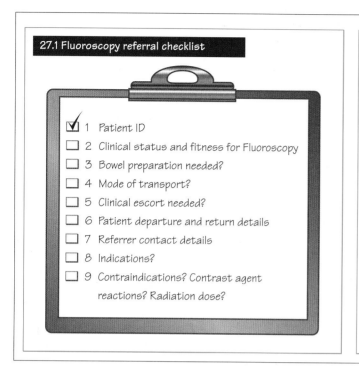

27.1 Fluoroscopy referral checklist

☑ 1 Patient ID
☐ 2 Clinical status and fitness for Fluoroscopy
☐ 3 Bowel preparation needed?
☐ 4 Mode of transport?
☐ 5 Clinical escort needed?
☐ 6 Patient departure and return details
☐ 7 Referrer contact details
☐ 8 Indications?
☐ 9 Contraindications? Contrast agent
       reactions? Radiation dose?

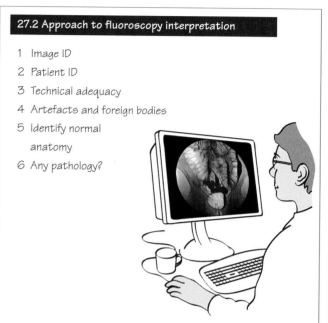

27.2 Approach to fluoroscopy interpretation

1 Image ID
2 Patient ID
3 Technical adequacy
4 Artefacts and foreign bodies
5 Identify normal
   anatomy
6 Any pathology?

Fluoroscopy referral checklist (see Chapter 7)

The imaging referral form is a legal document. The referrer has a legal responsibility to ensure that the correct and complete information is provided to the Imaging Department so that the patient is appropriately investigated and managed.

• **Patient identification:** The referrer must ensure that the Imaging Department receives the correct identification details of the patient to be investigated: full name, date of birth and hospital identification number are the essentials.

• **Clinical status:** The referrer must ensure that the patient's clinical condition and urgency with which the investigation is required are conveyed to the Imaging Department. Fluoroscopic investigations can take a long time and require the patient to be alert and co-operative. The referrer should discuss with the patient whether or not they are able and willing to undergo the investigation being requested, which can often be embarrassing for the patient (e.g. increased passing of flatus or incontinence with double contrast enema). If the patient is distracted by pain or other symptoms then an alternative investigation may be required. For many gastrointestinal fluoroscopic studies, bowel preparation in the form of starvation diet and/or laxatives are required in the days preceding the study to clear the alimentary canal of food products and faeculent material (Imaging Departments usually have individualised protocols).

• **Patient's mobility:** This is particularly relevant for fluoroscopic contrast studies where the patient may be required to be mobile (e.g. stand, roll over) in order to obtain the relevant images. If the patient is not able to undertake the necessary manoeuvres then an alternative investigation may be appropriate, e.g. CT colonography rather than barium enema. If there is doubt, the referrer should consult the radiologist.

• **Patient's location and travel details:** The patient's mobility also extends to their mode of transport to the Imaging Department. This includes the need for a clinical escort with patients requiring monitoring and therapeutic adjuncts such as supplementary oxygen or intravenous infusions. The points of departure and return and contact details must also be notified to the Imaging Department to ensure the patient is transferred safely and efficiently.

• **Indications:** Fluoroscopy has a variety of uses. The referral indication should always include a salient history and a specific question to be answered by fluoroscopy. In the context of fluoroscopic investigations of the GI tract, documentation with diagrams and explanation of any previous surgery or intervention is particularly helpful to avoid misinterpretation of unusual anatomy as pathology.

• **Contraindications:** The dose of ionising radiation from a fluoroscopic contrast study such as barium enema can be over 300 times that of a PA CXR. Important considerations include whether the patient has ever been given a contrast agent previously and, if so, was there any adverse reaction? Is the patient able to swallow the barium/water-soluble contrast agent? Has the patient been adequately prepared for the study (e.g. starvation diet, laxatives)? The referrer must therefore consider the clinical need and whether or not the result of the study will alter the patient's management.

Approach to interpreting fluoroscopic contrast studies

Correct interpretation of any radiographic image requires a systematic approach in order to ensure that all aspects of the investigation are assessed in a comprehensive manner and thus appropriate conclusions are reached. Fluoroscopic investigations are dynamic studies, which are performed in 'real time' and the images acquired depend on numerous factors including equipment, operator preference, and the patient's clinical condition and mobility. It is important that the images are labelled correctly at the time of acquisition. Interpretation of the investigation and the issuing of a report are therefore usually completed by the radiologist who undertook the study.

1 Identify the study and when it was conducted (see Chapter 2)
Video fluoroscopy, barium/water-soluble contrast swallow, barium/water-soluble contrast meal, small bowel meal, small bowel enema, double contrast barium enema or ERCP.

2 Identify the patient
Full name, sex, age and date of birth.

3 Technical adequacy
This should be assessed by the operator at the time of image acquisition and adequate views should be obtained to elucidate the relevant areas before the investigation is concluded. Considerations will vary depending upon the study being performed. In the case of a barium enema, important things to consider include adequate coverage (rectum to ileocaecal valve), correct amount of contrast, sufficient insufflation and ensuring that all areas are seen in double contrast. When reviewing the images it is important to ensure the images are correctly orientated to prevent misdiagnosis.

4 Artefacts and foreign bodies
Depending on the area covered by fluoroscopy, a variety of foreign bodies may be observed. The patient is asked to remove all jewellery and is dressed only in a gown. Consequently, there should be minimal external artefacts except for, for example, a colostomy bag.

Radio-opaque foreign bodies include: dental fillings; feeding tubes; false teeth; surgical clips; sternotomy wires; vascular coils; coronary stents; pacemaker/ICD; pacing wires; prosthetic heart valves; oesophageal stents; oesophageal and gastric bezoars; biliary, colonic or ureteric stents; urinary catheters; contraceptive coils; sterilisation clips and pessary rings; patient-inserted objects.

Identify normal anatomy of the GI tract

5 Pharynx
The pharynx is the part of the GI tract extending from the posterior oral and nasal cavities to the upper oesophagus and larynx. It is divided into the nasopharynx, oropharynx and hypopharynx. Only the oropharynx and hypopharynx are involved in swallowing.

6 Oesophagus
The oesophagus runs from the cricopharyngeus (C5, C6) superiorly to the gastro-oesophageal sphincter inferiorly. It is a compressible muscular tube, approximately 25 cm long, lying posterior to the trachea. It is usually observed during coordinated muscular contraction and should have a similar diameter throughout its length.

7 Stomach
The stomach is a J-shaped portion of the GI tract immediately inferior to the diaphragm. It begins at the gastro-oesophageal junction and ends at the pylorus, which connects the oesophagus to the duodenum. The stomach is anatomically divided into the cardia/fundus, body, antrum and pylorus. The rugae (folds of the stomach wall) are usually visible when the stomach wall is lined with contrast.

8 Small bowel
The small bowel is a tube stretching from the pyloric sphincter to the ileocaecal valve, connecting the stomach to the large bowel. It is subdivided into three segments; duodenum (25 cm), jejunum (2.5 m) and ileum (2 m). In order to provide the large surface area required for absorption it has many circular folds (valvulae conniventes), which in the normal individual can be appreciated on contrast-enhanced studies extending all the way across the lumen as they are contrast coated. The small bowel loops can sometimes be difficult to discern radiologically, as these loops may overlap and mimic the appearance of the large bowel. Patients are therefore appropriately manoeuvred to acquire the necessary views.

9 Large bowel
The large bowel extends approximately 1.5 m from the ileocaecal valve (a fold of mucous membrane) to the anus. It is approximately 6.5 cm in diameter and is indented by haustral folds. It is subdivided into four major segments; caecum, colon (ascending, descending, transverse and sigmoid), rectum and anal canal. The appendix is a narrow tapered tube of approximately 8 cm in length, and is attached to the lower portion of the caecum. When performing a large bowel enema it is important to visualise contrast agent refluxing either through the ileocaecal valve or into the appendix. This indicates that the contrast has reached the caecal pole and thereby ensures that the full length of the large bowel is coated for imaging.

28.1 Barium swallow – oesophageal cancer (barium is white)

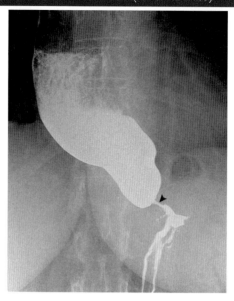

There is an irregular circumferential filling defect with 'shouldering' (*) from normal mucosa to abnormal mucosa. These are typical barium swallow features of oesophageal cancer and confirmed with endoscopy and biopsy

28.2 Barium swallow – achalasia (barium is white)

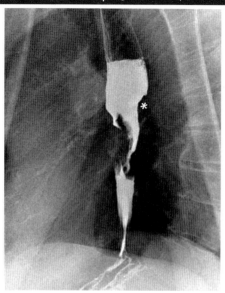

Normal peristalsis was absent in this patient. There is a narrowing of the lower oesophageal sphincter (LOS; arrowhead) and luminal dilatation above this level

28.3 Double-contrast barium enema (DCBE) – diverticular disease (barium is white)

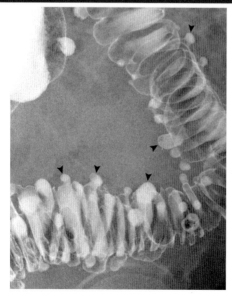

Numerous diverticula (arrowheads) in the sigmoid colon have filled with barium. The lumen is distended by pumping gas (CO_2 or air) into the rectum. No complications of diverticular disease such as stricturing are seen in this patient

28.4 Double-contrast barium enema (DCBE) – apple core lesion due to colorectal cancer (barium is white)

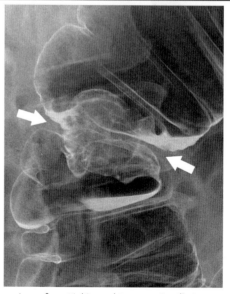

There is a circumferential irregular narrowing (between arrows) of the colonic lumen. This has the appearance of an apple core. Sigmoidoscopy and biopsy confirmed an adenocarcinoma

Oesophageal lesions

- **Webs and rings** – a web is a thin expansion of normal oesophageal tissue composed of mucosa and submucosa projecting into the lumen. A ring is a circumferential extension of normal oesophageal tissue containing mucosa, submucosa and muscle. Either can present with pain and dysphagia. Webs are commonest in the upper oesophagus and may be associated with Plummer-Vinson syndrome (web and iron deficiency anaemia) and can develop into carcinoma. Rings are more prevalent in the lower oesophagus, the commonest being the Schatzki ring (histologically a web since it contains only mucosa and submucosa). Barium swallow is an alternative option (to the first-line investigation of endoscopy) in patients presenting with dysphagia as well as those with a suspected web or ring.
- **Oesophageal stricture** – this is a fixed narrowing of the oesophageal lumen and may be classified into three groups.

  1 Intrinsic abnormalities – inflammation, fibrosis, neoplasia.

  2 Extrinsic abnormalities – compression (lymphadenopathy) or invasion (malignant tumour).

  3 Diseases affecting oesophageal peristalsis and/or gastro-oesophageal sphincter function (achalasia).

The causes of oesophageal stricture include gastro-oesophageal reflux disease (GORD), malignancy, caustic, radiation and iatrogenic damage. Fibrosis is the most common cause secondary to inflammation and neoplasm. Benign strictures are usually smoothly tapered concentric stenoses. Cancer of the oesophagus is adenocarcinoma secondary to Barrett's oesophagus in approximately 80–85% of cases and the remainder are squamous cell carcinomas. Oesophageal cancer rapidly invades local structures due to the absence of a serosal layer and has a very poor prognosis (five-year survival of 5%). It is usually appreciated radiographically as an asymmetric stricture, which is abrupt and eccentric, with an irregular ulcerated mucosa. Other patterns include polypoid (intraluminal filling defect), infiltrative and ulcerated mass.

- **Achalasia** – this is an idiopathic disorder characterised by a loss of ganglion cells in the myenteric plexus. This results in aperistalsis and raised pressure of the lower oesophageal sphincter (LOS), which fails to relax during swallowing. The oesophagus cannot empty and the patient is prone to dysphagia, regurgitation, halitosis and chest infections (secondary to aspiration). There is also an increased incidence of oesophageal cancer.

Small bowel lesions

- **Crohn's disease** (see Chapter 18) – fluoroscopic contrast studies of both the small and large bowel are useful for investigating Crohn's disease. Small bowel studies include small bowel meal and enema (see Chapter 2). Complications of Crohn's are common and best imaged using CT imaging or MRI.

Classic fluoroscopic features of Crohn's

- 'Rose thorn' ulcers (deep thorn-like indents in bowel wall)
- 'Cobblestoning' (linear ulcerations and fissures separating areas of raised oedematous mucosa)
- Widened and deformed valvulae conniventes
- Aperistalsis
- Luminal narrowing due to fibrotic strictures and thickened bowel wall especially of terminal ileum ('string sign of Kantor')
- Skip lesions (normal bowel between affected regions)
- Fistulae (between bowel loops or bowel and bladder/vagina)

Large bowel

- **Diverticular disease (diverticulosis)** – this is the presence of out-pouchings (diverticula) in the colon, which arise when the mucosa and submucosa bulges out through weak points in the bowel wall, often at vascular penetration points. It is related to hypertrophy of the muscular layers within the bowel wall and thought to arise secondary to raised intraluminal pressure and a 'western' low fibre diet. Many patients may be asymptomatic while others suffer from rectal bleeding, bloating, abdominal pain and altered bowel habit. Complications include diverticulitis, perforation, abscess and obstruction.
- **Colorectal cancer** – this is the second most common cause of cancer-related deaths in the developed world and both barium enema studies and colonoscopy are useful for primary diagnosis. CT colonography is now increasingly replacing the role of the barium enema. The rectum and sigmoid colon are the most common sites to be affected. Risk factors include advanced age, fatty diet, inflammatory bowel disease (principally ulcerative colitis) and genetic predisposition (hereditary polyposis and non-polyposis syndromes). Screening programmes for selected patients have led to early diagnosis and cure with resection. The disease is often silent but may present with abdominal pain, change in bowel habit and rectal bleeding. The work-up includes a staging CT with imaging of the chest, abdomen and pelvis.

Classic fluoroscopic features of oesophageal lesions

Webs/rings	Contrast-coated mucosal projection into lumen
Stricture	(Benign) contrast-coated short distal concentric luminal narrowing, tapered margins
	(Malignant) contrast-coated abrupt mucosal irregularity, prominent shoulders, tapered margins
Achalasia	Aperistalsis, luminal dilatation with standing column of contrast agent, air fluid level, 'beak' (tapered narrowing at the LOS), epiphrenic oesophageal diverticula (filled with contrast agent)

Classic fluoroscopic features of large bowel lesions (barium enema)

Diverticular disease
- Multiple smooth round bowel wall projections of varying size
- Common in sigmoid colon
- Bowel wall thickening may mimic carcinoma

Colorectal cancer
- 'Apple-core lesion' (irregular luminal narrowing with shouldering secondary to circumferential infiltration of wall)
- Polypoidal mass (intraluminal filling defect, often in caecum)

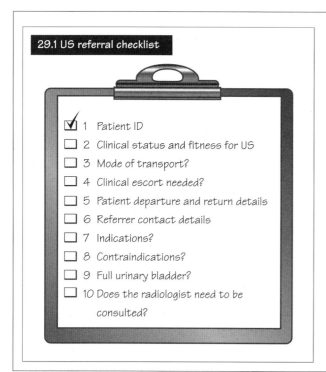

29.1 US referral checklist

☑ 1 Patient ID
☐ 2 Clinical status and fitness for US
☐ 3 Mode of transport?
☐ 4 Clinical escort needed?
☐ 5 Patient departure and return details
☐ 6 Referrer contact details
☐ 7 Indications?
☐ 8 Contraindications?
☐ 9 Full urinary bladder?
☐ 10 Does the radiologist need to be
        consulted?

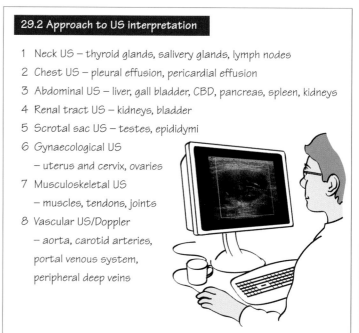

29.2 Approach to US interpretation

1 Neck US – thyroid glands, salivery glands, lymph nodes
2 Chest US – pleural effusion, pericardial effusion
3 Abdominal US – liver, gall bladder, CBD, pancreas, spleen, kidneys
4 Renal tract US – kidneys, bladder
5 Scrotal sac US – testes, epididymi
6 Gynaecological US
    – uterus and cervix, ovaries
7 Musculoskeletal US
    – muscles, tendons, joints
8 Vascular US/Doppler
    – aorta, carotid arteries,
    portal venous system,
    peripheral deep veins

US referral checklist (see Chapter 7)

The referrer carries the responsibility to ensure the correct and complete information is conveyed to the Imaging Department so that the patient is appropriately diagnosed and managed.

• **Patient identification:** The referrer must ensure that the Imaging Department receives the correct identification details of the patient to be investigated: full name, date of birth and hospital identification number are the essentials.

• **Clinical status:** The referrer must convey the patient's clinical condition and urgency of the referral to the Imaging Department.

• **Patient mobility:** Optimal images are obtained in slim patients using a sophisticated multifunctional departmental US machine. However, in some cases patients are too unwell to travel to the US department and thus US can be performed with a portable machine. US investigations using older portable machines are more limited in their imaging capacity and therefore may provide less detailed information compared with newer portable or departmental machines. The referrer must always consider the patient's clinical condition and refer for a departmental US study investigation if possible.

• **Patient location and travel details:** The need for a clinical escort should be conveyed. The points of departure and return, and contact details must also be notified to the Imaging Department to ensure the patient is transferred safely and efficiently.

• **Indications:** US often reveals a wide range of chest and abdominal pathology as well as subcutaneous, musculoskeletal and vascular pathology. US is also commonly used for interventional radiology procedures, e.g. biopsy and drainage of fluid collections. The referral indication should always include a salient history and a specific question to be answered by US.

• **Contraindications:** There are few contraindications for US, although image quality can be compromised by patient body habitus. For instance, in very obese patients with a thick layer of subcutaneous adipose tissue, image quality is impaired to the extent that the study is of very limited diagnostic benefit. In the case of US of the renal tract or gynaecological system, the referrer should ensure that the patient is advised to attend the US appointment with a full urinary bladder. This is because a fluid-filled bladder displaces structures that obscure the view (e.g. the bowel) and thereby provides a 'window' to see the pelvic structures more easily, particularly the ovaries. In interventional cases, the patient's coagulation status must be checked and any abnormalities corrected prior to the procedure. A recent coagulation profile should be communicated to the Imaging Department.

Approach to US interpretation

US is an excellent imaging investigation for muscles and tendons, visceral organs, reproductive organs, the fetus in utero, and other soft tissue structures. Image interpretation of US study investigations is primarily the remit of the radiologist or ultrasonographer. However, it is often helpful for clinicians to possess a basic understanding of how an US study is conducted and which structures can be seen. US images comprise areas of enhancement and shadowing. Tissues with higher than average attenuation (e.g. stones, gas) will cast a distal acoustic shadow and those with a lower than average attenuation (e.g. cyst) will cause distal acoustic enhancement. Common US imaging studies include:

• **Neck US** – this is used to visualise the *thyroid gland, salivary glands* and *lymph nodes*. The sequence usually begins with transverse images in the midline of the neck. This demonstrates the thyroid isthmus. Images are then taken of the thyroid lobes, followed by the lymph node chains, submandibular glands and parotid glands. Common cases for referral are those with a clinical history of a palpable face or neck lump (e.g. thyroid or salivary gland lesion).

• **Chest US** – this is performed to visualise the *chest wall* and *pleura*. Common cases for referral include eliciting the presence of a pleural effusion. Cardiologists also routinely use ultrasound (ECHO) to assess heart valves and ventricular size and function.

• **Abdominal US** – this is a common imaging investigation performed in the Imaging Department. US provides detailed images of the abdominal viscera including the *liver, gall bladder, pancreas, spleen* and *kidneys*. Detail of the bowel is less clearly seen due to the reflection of all sound waves by bowel gas. Moreover, gas-filled bowel often obscures other solid organ structures, particularly in the upper abdomen (e.g. pancreas). The abdominal US study may also include images of the full urinary bladder in the pelvis, followed by focused views of the left and right iliac fossae for intra-abdominal masses or other pathology. Commonest causes for referral include: right upper quadrant pain (e.g. gallstones, cholecystitis, hepatitis), jaundice (e.g. hepatitis, gallstones, tumour obstructing the biliary tree), right iliac fossa pain (e.g. appendicitis, ruptured ovarian cyst), left iliac fossa pain (e.g. diverticulitis, ruptured ovarian cyst), post-traumatic left upper quadrant pain (e.g. splenic injury). It should be highlighted that US cannot always reliably exclude certain pathologies, e.g. splenic injury. Therefore, patient management must be directed by the overall clinical suspicion in the face of a 'normal' US.

• **Renal tract US** – the renal tract US study focuses on both *kidneys* and the *urinary bladder*. The renal cortex, medulla and pelvi-calyceal systems are well visualised on US; however, the ureters themselves are not well seen. The study is best performed with a full urinary bladder, which helps differentiate it from other fluid collections in the pelvis and allows more accurate interpretation of any irregularities of the bladder wall. Images of the kidneys and bladder are acquired in two planes. Dimensions of the kidneys and pelvic outflow tract are normally measured and the bladder volume before and after micturition can also be obtained. The commonest cases for referral are patients with a clinical history of renal impairment and/or obstruction.

• **Testicular and epididymal US** – the testis and epididymis are superficial soft tissue structures and therefore very easily examined with US. US can also be used to identify an *inguinal hernia*. Doppler is applied to check the adequacy of vascular flow to the testes; however, US is not indicated in the scenario of suspected acute torsion. Such patients must be explored surgically at the earliest possible time. Common cases for referral are patients with a clinical history of a suspected lump or epididymo-orchitis.

• **Gynaecological US** – this is performed by radiologists, gynaecologists and ultrasonographers who may image using either transabdominal or transvaginal probes. It is imperative for patients to have a full urinary bladder for transabdominal US of the pelvis to optimise the imaging field. The *uterus, cervix* and *ovaries* can all be visualised. Common cases for referral are patients with pelvic pain (e.g. ovarian cyst), menorrhagia (e.g. fibroids, endometriosis) or post-menopausal bleeding.

• **Musculoskeletal US** – the superficial soft tissues of the musculoskeletal system i.e. *muscles, tendons* and *joints*, are well visualised on US. The bone surface may be seen but sound waves are reflected by cortical bone to the extent that no detail of the bone medulla can be appreciated. Musculoskeletal US is often performed by radiologists with a specific interest in musculoskeletal radiology due to the demands of complex anatomy. Common causes for referral include suspected muscle and tendon tears, joint effusions and soft tissue masses.

• **Vascular US/Doppler** – Doppler US is excellent for obtaining detailed information regarding *vascular flow*, using a non-invasive imaging technique. Colour Doppler can be applied to help interpret the direction of flow and flow velocities can be calculated. Common cases for referral include: carotid artery disease, aortic aneurysm, post-angiographic false femoral aneurysm, portal venous hypertension or occlusion and deep vein thrombosis.

• **Interventional US** – US-guided intervention is now routine in most hospitals. Common procedures include: *vascular access, biopsy* (e.g. liver, kidney, prostate, breast), *fine needle aspiration for cytology* (e.g. neck and breast lumps), *fluid aspiration and drain insertion* (e.g. pleural effusion, ascites, abscesses), *sealing of false femoral aneurysm* (procoagulant injection) and joint injections.

30.1 Liver metastases

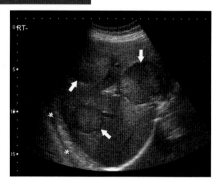

Multiple well-defined round lesions are seen in the liver (arrows). This was the first evidence of metastatic disease in this patient with a history of breast cancer. Depth in centimetres is shown down the side of the image. (*) diaphragm

30.2 Gallstone and cholecystitis

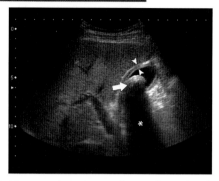

The gall bladder contains a large gallstone (arrow) with a distal acoustic shadow (*) (see Chapter 3). The gall bladder is thick-walled (arrowheads). These are the typical ultrasound features of cholecystitis

30.3 Renal cyst

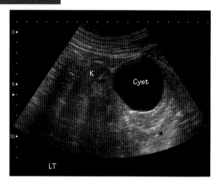

There is a cyst arising from the cortex of the kidney (K). This is causing acoustic enhancement artefact (*) (see Chapter 3). This cyst is simple in nature with a thin wall. The presence of features such as septation and calcification would be associated with an increased risk of malignancy

30.4 Lymph node biopsy

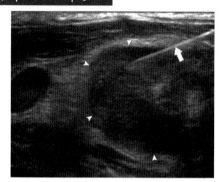

Ultrasound is an excellent tool for guided fine-needle aspiration (FNA). Here the FNA needle (arrow) can be seen passing into an enlarged lymph node (arrowheads). Fine movements and capillary action provide a small cytology sample which is examined microscopically

30.5 Testicular lesion

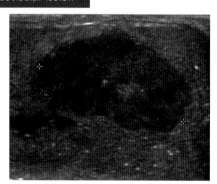

An ovoid irregular mass within the testis has been marked (crosses). Ultrasound is highly sensitive for detecting lesions in the testes. No preoperative FNA or biopsy was required for this lesion and the entire testis was removed. The lesion proved to be a seminoma, the commonest type of testicular malignancy

30.6 Bowel thickening: Crohn's disease

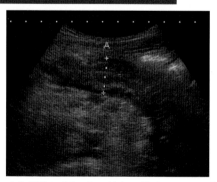

Measurement A (2.5 cm) is of a thick-walled segment of bowel thought to be the appendix in this patient who presented with right lower quadrant pain and tenderness. A subsequent CT demonstrated terminal ileitis. The normal appendix measures less than 10 mm but is thickened and non-compressible if inflamed

Liver lesions

The liver on US appears as a large solid structure lying in the right upper quadrant (RUQ) and has a uniform echotexture. It is supplied by the portal vein and hepatic artery, and is drained by the hepatic veins. Abnormalities of the liver include:
• *Metastatic disease* – these are focal areas of low, high or mixed echogenicity.
• *Cysts* – these are well-defined focal anechoic areas with distal acoustic enhancement.
• *Fatty infiltration* – the liver has patchy or geographic variation in echogenicity.
• *Cirrhosis* – the liver has an irregular or lobulated edge.
• *Biliary obstruction* – the common bile duct (CBD) is a tubular structure, which normally has a diameter of up to 6 mm. A dilated CBD is suggestive of biliary obstruction (e.g. due to gallstone, pancreatic tumour, cholangiocarcinoma).

Gall bladder lesions

The gall bladder appears as an anechoic saccular structure lying in the RUQ. Abnormalities of the gall bladder include:
• *Gallstones* – these are hyperechoic structures within the gall bladder, which cast distal anechoic shadows. Gallstones are gravity dependent and should therefore move on repositioning the patient. Non-gravity-dependent hyperechoic lesions include polyps arising from the gall bladder wall.
• *Acute cholecystitis* – the gall bladder wall is normally thin and uniform, measuring up to 3 mm in thickness. A thickened gall bladder wall with an anechoic perimeter of inflammatory fluid is highly suggestive of acute cholecystitis.

Pancreatic lesions

The pancreas appears as a long curved or comma-shaped homogeneous structure lying across the midline of the upper abdomen. The pancreatic head lies to the right of the midline, in the curve of the duodenal loop, and the tail points towards the splenic hilum in the left upper quadrant. Its echogenicity varies greatly with the age of the patient and the degree of fatty replacement. Views of the pancreas may be obscured if there is bowel gas casting shadows over it. Abnormalities of the pancreas include:
• *Pancreatic cancer* – a hypoechoic lesion at the pancreatic head is highly suspicious of a head of pancreas malignancy. This can impinge on the CBD and pancreatic duct causing proximal dilatation.
• *Acute pancreatitis* – a bulky pancreas with mixed echogenicity, often surrounded by anechoic inflammatory fluid is suggestive of acute pancreatitis.
• *Chronic pancreatitis* – the pancreas is relatively normal with flecks of hyperechoic microcalcifications.

Kidney lesions

The kidneys are seen in the coronal-oblique and axial planes and appear as solid structures in the flanks. The renal cortex has slightly lower echogenicity compared with the liver. The renal medulla is more hypoechoic compared with the liver and the renal sinus (proximal collecting system and renal fat) is comparatively hyperechoic. The pelvi-calyceal system contains urine and is therefore anechoic, however in many cases the calyces may only be seen if dilated. Abnormalities of the kidney include:
• *Cysts* – these are well-defined, thin-walled, anechoic, spherical structures arising from the renal cortex with distal acoustic enhancement. Renal cysts can be of any size; however, if they become septated or more complex in architecture, the concern for malignant change should be raised.
• *Renal outflow obstruction (hydronephrosis)* – a dilated anechoic pelvi-calyceal system may be due to a distal urinary calculus or tumour.
• *Chronic renal disease* – the cortex is thin and lobulated.

Pleural effusion (see Chapter 12)

Pleural effusions are best seen with the patient sat upright so that the fluid collects above the hemidiaphragms. Pleural effusions appear as anechoic areas, but if the architecture is more complex it may suggest an empyema. Diffuse pleural thickening may suggest mesothelioma or pleural metastases. US is often used to mark the optimum site to drain a pleural effusion. It should be remembered that since fluid is gravity dependent, the site marked is only accurate if the chest drain is inserted with the patient in the same position as when the site was marked.

Neck lumps

The thyroid and salivary glands on US are homogeneous in echotexture and have mid-level echogenicity. The classic appearance of a normal lymph node is oval, well-defined, hypoechoic, homogeneous, and with a hyperechoic central hilum. If these features are absent then malignant infiltration should be considered. Abnormalities of the thyroid and salivary glands include:
• *Salivary gland neoplasm* – well-defined hypoechoic masses within the salivary glands are usually benign (e.g. pleomorphic adenoma, Warthin's tumour). Less well-defined masses, which breach anatomic boundaries and have deranged vasculature, raise the possibility of malignant lesions (e.g. squamous cell carcinoma). US cannot definitively distinguish between these lesions and therefore FNAC is routinely performed.
• *Thyroid cancer* – these are usually solid or complex lesions in the thyroid gland.
• *Colloid nodules* – these are anechoic thin-walled circular strictures in the thyroid gland.

Scrotal lumps

The testes have a fine homogeneous texture. The epididymi are well seen at the superior and inferior testicular poles. They are recognised by their mid-level echogenicity with anechoic tubules and vessels. US is highly sensitive for scrotal lumps and is therefore the best imaging method for such lesions. Abnormalities of the scrotum include:
• *Testicular cancer* – most focal abnormalities within the testicular parenchyma should be regarded as malignant until proven otherwise.
• *Epididymal cysts* – these are well-defined, thin-walled, anechoic, circular structures in the epididymis.
• *Hydrocoele* – the testis is surrounded by anechoic fluid.

Appendicitis

The role of US in the management of appendicitis is contentious as visualisation of the appendix is variable. Appendicitis has traditionally been a clinical diagnosis but US may help to assess an appendix mass or abscess. The inflamed appendix, when seen, appears as a thick-walled, blind-ending, non-compressible tubular structure lying in the right iliac fossa. There may also be a surrounding anechoic area, representing inflammatory fluid.

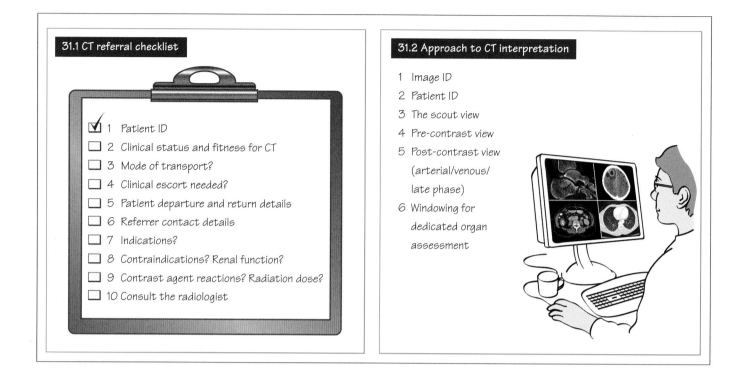

31.1 CT referral checklist

- ☑ 1 Patient ID
- ☐ 2 Clinical status and fitness for CT
- ☐ 3 Mode of transport?
- ☐ 4 Clinical escort needed?
- ☐ 5 Patient departure and return details
- ☐ 6 Referrer contact details
- ☐ 7 Indications?
- ☐ 8 Contraindications? Renal function?
- ☐ 9 Contrast agent reactions? Radiation dose?
- ☐ 10 Consult the radiologist

31.2 Approach to CT interpretation

1 Image ID
2 Patient ID
3 The scout view
4 Pre-contrast view
5 Post-contrast view (arterial/venous/ late phase)
6 Windowing for dedicated organ assessment

CT referral checklist (see Chapter 7)

The imaging referral form is a legal document. The referrer carries the responsibility to ensure the correct and complete information is conveyed to the Imaging Department so that the patient is appropriately diagnosed and managed.

• **Patient identification:** The referrer must ensure that the Imaging Department receives the correct identification details of the patient to be investigated: full name, date of birth and hospital identification number are the essentials.

• **Clinical status:** The referrer must convey the patient's clinical condition and urgency of the referral to the Imaging Department. CT has now become a mainstay for definitive diagnosis in both the emergency and elective setting.

• **Patient mobility:** CT can be used to image the very well to the very sickest of patients. However, in unstable patients the clinical risk of transferring the patient to the CT scanner must be weighed up against the clinical urgency for diagnostic information for management planning or therapeutic intervention. This avoids the CT scanner being labelled the 'doughnut of death' by reducing the risk of patients suffering a cardiac arrest on the CT table. The referrer must also confirm the CT table's maximum licensed weight with the scanning radiographer, before referring patients with a high body mass index.

• **Patient location and travel details:** The need for a clinical escort should be conveyed and the points of departure and return and contact details must also be notified to the Imaging Department to ensure the patient is transferred safely and efficiently. For multi-trauma patients or patients from the intensive care unit, an anaesthetist or intensive care physician escort may well be required.

• **Indications:** Multi-detector CT can now reveal a huge range of pathology in most parts of the body. CT is also commonly used for interventional radiology procedures, e.g. biopsy and drainage of fluid collections. The referral indication should always include a salient history and a specific question to be answered by CT.

• **Contraindications:** The primary contraindications for CT relate to the use of intravenous contrast agents and levels of radiation exposure (see Chapter 6). In those patients who have a history of adverse reactions to iodinated contrast agents and those with poor renal function, CT imaging with intravenous contrast agents is generally contraindicated. In some cases, however, the clinical need may outweigh the clinical risk and these cases should be discussed with the radiologist performing the procedure. In all cases therefore, where intravenous contrast is likely to be used, the patient's renal function should be checked before CT imaging and the eGFR communicated to the Imaging Department. In those patients who have had multiple previous CT imaging or are likely to go on to have subsequent CT imaging, the total radiation dose must be considered to reduce the risk of long-term adverse effects of radiation. In such cases, alternative lower-radiation dose diagnostic imaging techniques, or those requiring no radiation, e.g. MRI or US, should be considered. In interventional radiology or biopsy cases, the patient's coagulation status must be checked and correction of clotting abnormalities may be necessary before the procedure. For this reason, the most recent coagulation profile should be communicated to the Imaging Department.

Approach to CT interpretation

Plain X-ray imaging is limited by its two-dimensional representation of three-dimensional structures. Modern CT imaging now allows the acquired X-ray data to be reformatted into volumetric three-dimensional representations.

Different anatomical structures have different inherent densities and therefore different characteristic appearances on CT. The Hounsfield units (HU) of the principal components are relative to the density of air and water, −1000 and 0 respectively. (Other figures in the table below are approximate.)

CT densities

• Air	−1000 HU
• Fat	−50 to −100 HU
• Water	0 HU
• Muscle	+10 to +40 HU
• Visceral organs	+20 to +40 HU
• Blood	+40 HU
• Bone	+1000 HU

Advances in CT imaging permit high resolution imaging for detailed evaluation of virtually all parts of the body. CT imaging is now the gold standard in the diagnosis of many diseases and it is increasingly being investigated as a screening tool for early detection, e.g. lung cancer. Images are acquired in the transverse/axial plane and interpretation therefore relies on a thorough understanding of topographical cross-sectional anatomy and normal variants. These images are viewed as if from below and looking cranially. Although coronal and sagittal reformatted images are very helpful, axial images are often the most useful for diagnostic purposes. A systematic approach to viewing and assessing an axial CT image series is therefore vital to identify normal structures and anatomical variants, as well as avoiding missing expected and unexpected pathology.

The scout view

A 'scout view' image is acquired before the main scan in order to plan for complete coverage of the area of interest. The scout view is also sometimes useful to elicit any gross abnormality before assessing the image series more thoroughly. The subsequent images are acquired into a three-dimensional dataset, which can be further manipulated and reformatted.

High resolution CT

If higher resolution images are necessary, e.g. in lung imaging, high resolution CT (HRCT) may be performed. This involves acquiring data in thin slices with an interslice space of approximately 1–2 cm. As a result, fine detail of these representative slices can be determined. Small abnormalities that only lie within the interslice spaces, however, may not be included. HRCT is therefore used to diagnose and monitor diffuse structural lung disease such as pulmonary fibrosis but is not used for the detection of small focal abnormalities.

Imaging with contrast agent enhancement

The use of a water-soluble intravenous contrast agent can significantly enhance the quality of CT imaging and aid the diagnostic process in many clinical settings. The timing of the acquisition of images post-administration of the contrast agent is often very important. If images are obtained after approximately 30 seconds, the contrast agent will be mainly circulating in the arterial system and is therefore known as the arterial phase. If CT images of the abdomen are obtained at approximately 60 seconds, the contrast agent will be mainly circulating in the portal venous system and this is therefore known as the portal venous phase. CT angiography is performed in the arterial phase to capture the contrast agent in the systemic arterial circulation. The acquisition of CT images may be triggered by detection of the contrast agent reaching a particular vessel. A CT pulmonary angiogram, for example, is triggered when the contrast agent reaches either the right atrium or the main pulmonary artery. Timing is particularly important in this setting, as circulation in patients with suspected pulmonary embolism is variable due to large variations in cardiac output. Incorrect timing may risk missing the diagnosis. Imaging of the abdomen, on the other hand, is usually performed in the portal venous phase to capture the contrast agent in the portal venous circulation, which supplies the liver. In many cases, however, dual imaging (arterial and portal venous), triphasic imaging (pre-contrast, arterial and portal), or even four-phase imaging (triphasic and delayed) is performed to elicit certain specific pathologies.

Opacification of the GI tract with an oral and/or rectal contrast agent is common practice for studies of the abdomen and pelvis. The oral agent is typically given one hour before imaging but rectal contrast is usually administered in the CT suite itself. A 'negative' oral contrast agent (e.g. water) is commonly used for stomach and proximal small bowel imaging studies. For large bowel imaging studies, a 'positive' contrast agent (e.g. an iodine-based solution) is usually used. Gas in the form of air or carbon dioxide can also be administered rectally to provide double contrast imaging, e.g. CT colonography.

Windowing

The spectrum of Hounsfield unit densities in any axial image is often very large due to the wide range of structures in the field of view. It is possible however to view a defined range or 'window' of Hounsfield units which allows resolution of increased numbers of shades of grey, providing greater specificity of detail to different structures. Various window ranges are centred on the Hounsfield unit values of important structures (lungs, soft tissues, bone, liver). It is therefore important to evaluate specific individual structures in their optimised window setting. This is achieved using the same CT data but with software manipulation.

32.1 Soft tissue windows: heart

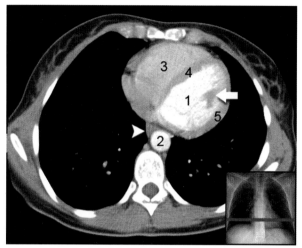

Intravenous contrast is seen in the left ventricle (1) and descending aorta (2). Structures of the heart such as the right ventricle (3), intraventricular septum (4), left ventricular free wall (5) and papillary muscles (arrow) are clearly seen. The tissue adjacent to the aorta is the oesophagus (arrowheads)

32.2 Lung windows: just above carina

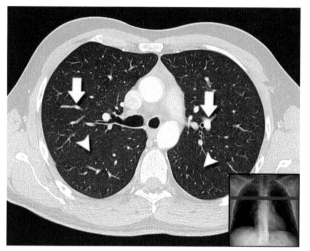

Here the major fissures can be seen on both sides (arrowheads). The branches of the pulmonary vessels are seen (arrows) which make up the lung markings on a plain CXR

32.3 Soft tissue windows: at carina

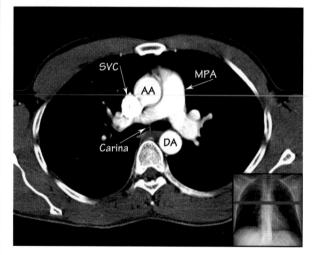

At the level of the carina the main pulmonary artery (MPA) is seen to branch into left and right main pulmonary arteries. The superior vena cava (SVC) lies immediately above the right atrium. The ascending aorta (AA) arches over the pulmonary vessels and major bronchi to join the descending aorta (DA)

32.4 Lung windows: through diaphragm

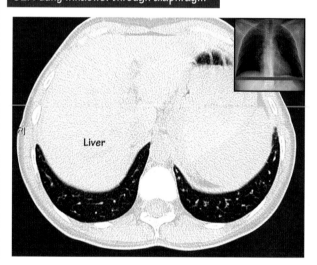

Crescents of lung tissue are seen within the posterior recess of the chest cavity. These parts of the lungs are not easily visible on plain CXR. Soft tissues of the abdomen, such as the liver, are visible immediately below the diaphragm but no detail is provided when viewing with lung window settings

Chest anatomy seen on CT

CT is superior to plain X-ray imaging in demonstrating the anatomical structures of the chest. Some structures invisible on CXR (e.g. oesophagus) are clearly seen on CT and other structures are seen with far greater detail (e.g. heart, with separation of all chambers and myocardium from pericardium). The vessels of the chest including the aorta, great vessels of the neck, pulmonary vessels and even the coronary vessels are easily appreciated. Fine detail of lung structure is determined on CT and soft tissue planes are readily distinguished. Certain important anatomical structures however remain difficult to see (e.g. lymphatic system including the thoracic duct). Nerves such as the phrenic, vagus and costal nerves are not conspicuous on CT. In most cases, viewing of image data is in two different window settings (soft tissue and lung) and the adjustment of software settings can improve the visual perception of certain tissues, such as bone. Important structures visible on axial CT of the chest include:

Peripheral soft tissue structures

• *Subcutaneous fat* – this is seen as a rim of very low-density soft tissue surrounding the rib cage.
• *Breast tissue* – this lies in the anterior chest wall, is most often seen continuous with subcutaneous fat, and contains various components of higher density glandular tissue.
• *Muscles* – these are seen as smooth mid-density structures in the chest wall and paraspinal regions, arising from and inserting into bone.
• *Lymph nodes* – these typically appear as small bean-shaped, mid-density soft tissue structures. They are often seen in the central, supraclavicular, axillary and mediastinal regions. They normally measure less than 1 cm in short axis diameter and may be seen to have a central fatty low-density hilum.
• *Diaphragm* – this is an imperceptibly thin layer, separating the lungs from the abdominal organs. The thick crura are seen arising posteriorly from the upper lumbar vertebrae.

Central soft tissue structures

• *Heart* – this is a large central mid-density soft tissue structure. The right atrium and ventricle lie anteriorly and to the right of the left atrium and ventricle, which lie posteriorly. The valves and septa are also visualised. The coronary arteries are seen arising from the aortic root and running over the heart's surface in the epicardial fat. The pericardium is seen as a thin (1–2 mm) dense soft tissue layer encasing the heart but separated from it by a thin layer of epicardial fat.
• *Aorta* – this is a thick-walled tubular structure, arising from the left ventricle. It can then be mapped as it ascends, arches posteriorly to the left, and descends down the left side of the mediastinum decreasing in diameter until it pierces the diaphragm. (Normal diameter is <4 cm.)
• *SVC* – this is a tubular structure, descending to the right of the midline and into the right atrium. Its diameter can vary (1–2.5 cm).
• *Pulmonary arteries* – the pulmonary trunk (2.5 cm diameter) arises from the right ventricle and lies anterior to the ascending aorta. As the pulmonary trunk ascends, it twists around the left side of the

ascending aorta to lie behind it and beneath the aortic arch. At this point the pulmonary trunk bifurcates into the left and right pulmonary arteries, the right pulmonary artery passing in front of the right main bronchus and the left passing over the top and posterior to the left main bronchus. This accounts for the main asymmetry of the hilar structures seen on normal CXR. The pulmonary arteries accompany their respective bronchus as they branch into the pulmonary tree.
• *Pulmonary veins* – these are tubular structures, flowing into the left atrium. The upper lobe pulmonary veins are relatively vertical and pass anterior to the bronchi. The lower lobe pulmonary veins are relatively horizontal and pass in a plane posterior to the bronchi.
• *Azygos vein* – this is a small tubular structure, passing vertically on the right side in the posterior mediastinum, adjacent to the oesophagus. At the level of T4, it arches anteriorly to drain into the SVC.
• *Hemiazygos vein* – this is a small tubular structure, passing in the posterior mediastinum along the left side of the aorta, and crossing behind it to drain into the azygos vein at T8 level.
• *Oesophagus* – this is a tubular structure, descending in the posterior mediastinum behind the trachea. It may contain air or food.
• *Lymph nodes* – As in the periphery, these usually appear as well-defined bean-shaped soft tissue structures (<1 cm short axis diameter) with a low-density central fatty hilum. There are several groups of central lymph nodes, which are named according to their location (e.g. paratracheal, paraaortic, paraoesophageal, hilar, mediastinal).

Lungs and airways

• *Trachea* – this is a thin-walled midline air-filled tubular structure with a diameter of approximately 1.5–2 cm. The trachea descends almost vertically in the mediastinum, running anterior to the oesophagus and bifurcates into the left and right main bronchi at the carina (approximately T5 level).
• *Main bronchi* – these air-filled tubular structures descend obliquely into their respective lungs. The right main bronchus is wider, shorter and more vertical than the left.
• *Lungs* – the air-filled lungs appear as very low-density tissues and the higher density pulmonary vascular network comprises the lung markings. The fissures can often be seen separating the lobes.
• *Pleura* – these are not usually distinguished from structures of the thoracic wall on CT imaging unless abnormally thickened, however the pleura of the fissures of each lung can often be seen clearly (Figure 32.2).

Bones

For CT imaging of the chest, the arms are extended above the head and the shoulders are incorporated. The visible bones include:
• *Spine* – lower cervical vertebrae to upper lumbar vertebrae.
• *Sternum.*
• *Ribs.*
• *Clavicles.*
• *Scapulae.*
• *Proximal left and right humerus.*

33.1 Pneumonia (lung windows)

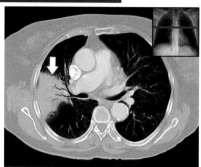

The wedge-shaped segment of high density (arrow) is consolidation. There are several branching airways which have remained open (black) within surrounding small airways that are full of pus (grey). This phenomenon is known as 'air bronchogram' and is a characteristic finding of consolidation of the lung

33.2 Pleural effusion (soft tissue windows)

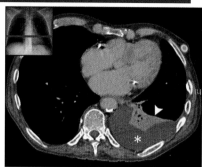

The patient is lying down for the scan and so the effusion appears as a crescent of fluid collected in the posterior pleural space (*). As is often seen with pleural effusions there is an area of atelectasis (collapse) seen at its upper surface (arrowhead)

33.3 Pneumothorax (lung windows)

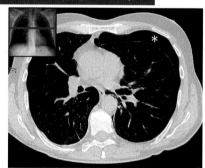

There is a large crescentic rim of air (*) seen at the front of the left pleural space. It has collected here because the patient is lying down whereas on an erect CXR it would collect at the lung apex. Note the density (blackness) of the air collection is exactly the same as the air outside the chest wall

33.4 Emphysema (lung windows)

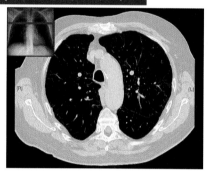

This patient has marked bullous emphysema. Holes throughout the lung parenchyma distort the pulmonary vessels. This mainly affects the upper parts of the lungs in smoking-related cases. The shape of the chest is also changed due to lung hyperexpansion such that the chest is wider than normal from front to back

33.5 Bronchiectasis (lung windows)

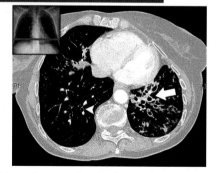

In the left lung there is a 'bunch of grapes' appearance (arrow) which indicates a localised area of severe bronchiectasis. The airways are bigger than their accompanying vessels. This can also be seen in the right lung (arrowhead) but is much less severe

33.6 Fibrosis (HRCT lung windows)

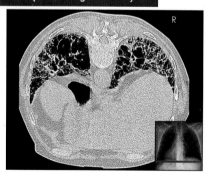

The patient has been scanned in the prone position. There are 'honeycomb' holes in the lung parenchyma. Unlike emphysema these holes have thick walls

Pneumonia

Pneumonia is an acute infection of the lower respiratory tract. Incidence is 1–3 per 1000 in the UK and typically presents in the elderly, young and immunocompromised. The pathogens invade the cells of the respiratory tract and/or the spaces around them, causing cell death and triggering an immune response that stimulates white blood cells to mount a defence. The inflammatory response causes fluid leakage into the alveoli, impairing gaseous exchange and leading to breathlessness, productive cough and pyrexia.

• **Community acquired pneumonia** is the commonest type, most often caused by *Streptococcus pneumoniae* followed by *Haemophilus influenzae*, *Mycoplasma pneumoniae* and *Staphylococcus aureus*. Viruses account for roughly 15%.

• **Nosocomial pneumonia** is acquired post 48 hours after admission to hospital and commonly caused by gram-negative *Enterobacteria*, *Staphylococcus aureus* and *Pseudomonas*.

• **Aspiration pneumonia** can occur in patients with stroke, reduced consciousness, myasthenia, bulbar palsies and oesophageal disease.

Classic CT features of pneumonia

- Air-space consolidation in a lobar distribution
- Small pleural effusion
- Ground glass attenuation with air bronchograms
- Centrilobar nodules
- Bronchial wall thickening
- Centrilobar branching structures

Pleural effusion (see Chapter 12)

Classic CT features of pleural effusion

- Crescent shaped, water attenuation in dependent areas
- Fluid accumulates posteriorly in costophrenic sulcus in supine position and extends apico-anteriorly
- Upward concave configuration of lung–effusion interface due to lung recoil
- Pleural thickening and enhancement suggests underlying inflammation, infection or neoplasm

Bronchiectasis

Bronchiectasis occurs secondary to chronic infection or obstruction of the central airways and is characterised by irreversible dilatation of part of the bronchial tree. This causes airflow obstruction and impaired clearance of mucus, and often affects patients with cystic fibrosis, Kartagener's syndrome, TB and HIV. Common pathogens causing infection include *H. influenzae*, *S. pneumoniae*, *Staph. aureus* and *Pseudomonas*. Impaired ciliary clearance of mucus and dilatation of the bronchial tree predisposes to infection. Lung damage ensues following recurrent infections, increasing the susceptibility to further infection.

Classic CT features of bronchiectasis

- Dilated airways: airways larger than their accompanying vessels with a 'signet ring' appearance; 'grape-like clusters' in more severely affected areas
- Bronchial wall thickening

Pneumothorax (see Chapter 13)

Classic CT features of pneumothorax

- Air between lung and chest wall in non-dependent areas
- Underlying causes, e.g. emphysema/bullae, chest wall trauma, apical fibrosis and consolidation

Chronic obstructive pulmonary disease (COPD)

COPD is a chronic, progressive lung disorder, characterised by chronic bronchitis, emphysema and airways obstruction ($\downarrow$FEV$_1$, $\downarrow$FEV$_1$/FVC). The commonest cause is tobacco smoking. Alpha-1-antitrypsin deficiency is a rare cause.

• **Chronic bronchitis** is defined as a *productive cough for three months of a year, for two consecutive years*. Increased goblet cell activity results in excess mucous secretions causing airway obstruction.

• **Emphysema** is defined as enlargement of the air spaces distal to the terminal bronchioles with wall destruction. The enlarged alveoli lead to reduced surface area available for gaseous exchange. This is usually diagnosed on CT.

Classic CT features of emphysema

- Multiple lucencies of destroyed parenchyma
- Possible associated pneumothorax

Pulmonary fibrosis

Pulmonary fibrosis is a disease characterised by scarring of the alveoli and interstitial tissue of the lungs. The causes include sarcoidosis, occupational lung disease (e.g. farmer's lung), asbestosis, drugs, radiotherapy and TB. In most cases, however, the cause is idiopathic. Chronic interstitial inflammation or some other trigger activates the proliferation of fibroblasts leading to pulmonary fibrosis and tissue destruction.

Classic CT features of fibrosis

- Peripheral and subpleural intralobular septal thickening
- Loss in lung volume
- Honeycombing
- Traction bronchiectasis

34.1 Primary lung cancer (soft tissue windows)

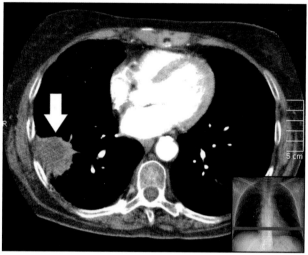

A large spiculated mass is seen adjacent to the pleura in the posterior right lung (arrow). This was biopsied under CT guidance and shown to be a squamous cell carcinoma

34.2 Lung metastases (lung windows)

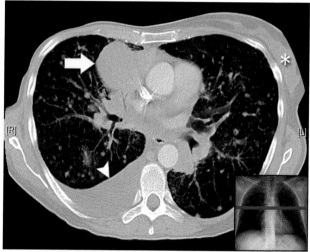

This patient had a known history of breast cancer. Note the right breast is absent following mastectomy. The normal left breast tissue is marked (*). There are multiple small lung nodules that are metastatic deposits. There is also a large round mass next to the right side of the heart (arrow) and a pleural effusion (arrowhead) seen posteriorly in the chest on the right

34.3 Mediastinal lymphadenopathy (soft tissue windows)

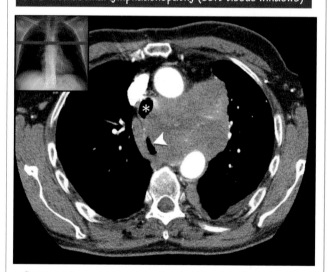

There is a large confluent mediastinal lymph node mass. This is located between the aortic arch and the pulmonary artery (not shown) in a space known as the aorto-pulmonary window. The mass was found to be a lung cancer and is causing deviation of the trachea (*) and oesophagus (arrowhead) to the right

34.4 Mesothelioma (soft tissue windows)

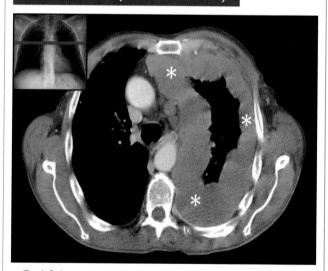

The left lung is encased in grossly thickened pleura (*). This patient has end-stage mesothelioma. The tumour mass has started to deviate the mediastinal structures towards the other side of the chest

Lung cancer (see Chapter 14)

A lung cancer may be suspected from appearances on CXR (e.g. a focal mass or lobar collapse) or from the clinical history (e.g. cough and weight loss in a smoker). However, further imaging with CT is required for TNM (tumour, nodes, metastases) staging and for planning of procedures such as biopsy and surgery.

- **Staging** of lung cancer is determined by the TNM status.
  - T – Tumour size, position and invasion of adjacent structures.
  - N – Lymph node number and position.
  - M – Metastatic disease. Common sites for metastasis include the adrenal glands and liver. Other sites may also be imaged depending on the clinical suspicion (e.g. CT of the brain or NM bone scan).
- **Biopsy planning** of a lung cancer is now routinely performed by CT to determine the optimum approach to obtain adequate tissue samples for histological diagnosis and tumour grading. A central peribronchial lesion may be relatively easily reached via bronchoscopy, whereas a peripheral lung lesion is often more readily accessible under CT or fluoroscopic guidance.

Classic CT features of lung cancer

- Spiculated or lobulated lung nodule or mass
- Possible airway obstruction causing lobar collapse
- Enlarged mediastinal lymph nodes (may be the dominant feature, especially in small cell lung cancer)
- Pleural effusion
- Invasion of thoracic wall or rib destruction

Mediastinal lymph node enlargement

(see Chapter 14)

CT is commonly indicated for investigating suspected mediastinal lymphadenopathy. It allows for more accurate localisation of enlarged lymph nodes (usually taken as >1 cm in their short axis diameter), determination of their morphology, and further patterns of lung disease to identify the root cause, e.g. lung masses, infection.

Classic CT features of lymph node involvement

- Enlargement >1 cm (short axis diameter)
- Compression of adjacent structures if large
- Underlying lung pathology, e.g. infection, mass, fibrosis

Mesothelioma

Mesothelioma is a cancer of the mesothelial membrane (e.g. the pleura, pericardium, peritoneum). The commonest site is the pleura and it is related to previous asbestos exposure. The symptoms, however, including shortness of breath, cough and chest pain, may not appear for 20 to 50 years after the exposure. There is frequently an associated pleural effusion at presentation. CXR and CT are the primary diagnostic imaging tools. Histological diagnosis can be achieved by CT-guided tissue biopsy and cytology obtained from US-guided aspiration of a malignant pleural effusion. If mesothelioma is suspected, these procedures should be performed with precaution, as there is high risk of tumour spreading (seeding) along the percutaneous needle track. This risk may be reduced by administering radiotherapy to the biopsy area.

Classic CT features of mesothelioma

- Unilateral pleural effusion
- Nodular pleural thickening including the mediastinal and interlobular fissural surfaces
- Contraction/volume loss of affected hemithorax

Aortic dissection (see Chapter 41)

Aortic dissection is a tear in the inner wall of the aorta, which then permits blood to flow between the layers of the vessel wall. A tear of the inner layer (tunica intima) of the aortic wall allows high-pressure aortic blood to force its way through the wall layers, causing them to separate or dissect away from the outer layer (tunica adventitia). This creates a second aortic lumen, known as a false lumen, which can then propagate along the aorta in a distal or proximal direction. Patients usually present with sudden onset of severe chest and/or back pain, which may progress if the dissection expands. The risk factors for aortic dissection include hypertension, Marfan's and Ehlers Danlos syndromes. Aortic dissection *is a surgical emergency* and early diagnosis is therefore essential. If the patient's clinical condition allows, CT arteriography is the investigation of choice, where advanced reformatting techniques can provide multiplanar images to assist surgical planning.

Classic CT features of aortic dissection

- A linear region of low attenuation within the lumen of the aorta on contrast-enhanced CT represents the torn intimal flap
- Associated features, e.g. aneurysm, thrombus within aortic lumen, haemorrhage, tamponade (liquid in the pericardial sac)

Pulmonary embolism (see Chapter 41)

Pulmonary embolism (PE) is the obstruction of a vessel in the pulmonary arterial tree by an embolus, most commonly originating from a deep venous thrombus. Presenting symptoms and signs include tachycardia, tachypnoea, shortness of breath, pleuritic chest pain, haemoptysis, haemodynamic compromise and collapse. Patients at increased risk include those who have compromised mobility, hypercoagulable states, malignancy, or are post trauma or surgery. CXR is the first-line investigation for patients with shortness of breath and is useful in determining further management decisions if PE is suspected. If the CXR is normal then ventilation-perfusion imaging is often the next investigation of choice. If the CXR is abnormal and the clinical suspicion remains high, dedicated imaging of the pulmonary arterial tree by a CT pulmonary angiogram (CTPA) is indicated.

Classic CTPA features of PE

- Intraluminal filling defect(s) in pulmonary arterial tree
- Enlargement of the main pulmonary artery and right atrium due to right heart strain
- Wedge lung infarction
- Hypoperfusion of lung in distribution of the occluded vessel
- Chronic PE may lead to vessels that are smaller than comparative patent vessels

35.1 CT Abdomen: upper abdomen

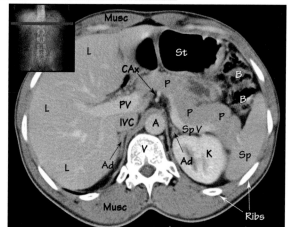

35.2 CT Abdomen: mid-abdomen

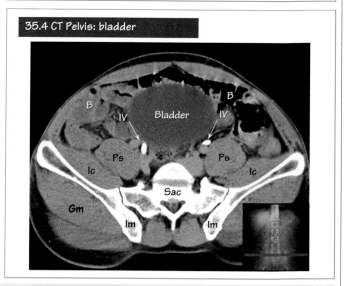

35.3 CT Abdomen: lower abdomen

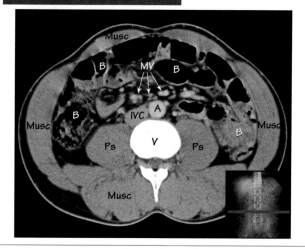

35.4 CT Pelvis: bladder

Key			
A – Aorta	Iv – Iliac vessels	Ps – Psoas muscle
Ad – Adrenal gland	IVC – Inferior vena cava	PV – Portal vein
B – Bowel	K – Kidney	Sac – Sacrum
CAx – Coeliac axis/trunk	L – Liver	Sp – Spleen
Gm – Gluteus muscles	Musc – Muscles of abdomen and back	SpV – Splenic vein
Ic – Iliacus muscle	MV – Mesenteric vessels	St – Stomach
Im – Ilium	P – Pancreas	U – Ureter
		V – Vertebral body

Abdominal anatomy seen on CT

CT is superior to plain X-ray imaging in demonstrating abdominal anatomy. Data is usually acquired during the portal venous phase of contrast agent enhancement (approximately 60–70 seconds post-injection) to optimise delineation of the liver, which derives its primary supply from the portal vein. Important structures visible on abdominal CT include:

- *Stomach* – this left upper quadrant hollow structure extends across the epigastrium. It is divided into the fundus, body, antrum and pylorus, and its blood supply is derived from the coeliac trunk.
- *Small bowel* – this very long central abdominal meandering tubular structure comprises the duodenum, jejunum and ileum. The duodenum is split into four parts with the first, second and third parts forming a C-loop around the pancreatic head. The second, third and fourth parts are retroperitoneal. The jejunum runs for approximately 2.5 m before transitioning into the ileum for 2 m. The jejunum and ileum are suspended by mesentery.
- *Large bowel* – this peripheral abdominal long tubular structure is divided into the caecum, ascending colon (right-sided retroperitoneal ascent to hepatic flexure), transverse colon (transverse intraperitoneal course from hepatic to splenic flexure and suspended by transverse mesocolon), descending colon (left-sided retroperitoneal descent from splenic flexure to sigmoid colon) and sigmoid colon (in the upper pelvis and attached by sigmoid mesocolon). At the ileocaecal junction lies the ileocaecal valve. The appendix is a blind-ending tubular structure originating 2–3 cm inferior to the ileocaecal valve and has a variable position.
- *Rectum* – this retroperitoneal hollow structure lies behind the bladder in males and behind the uterus and vagina in females.
- *Liver* – this large right upper quadrant solid structure is made up of four lobes (right, left, caudate and quadrate) or eight segments. It is supplied by the portal vein and common hepatic artery and drained by the right, middle and left hepatic veins into the IVC.
- *Gall bladder* – this saccular structure lies between the liver's right and quadrate lobes and stores bile. It is supplied by the cystic artery and connects to the common hepatic duct via the cystic duct, thereby forming the common bile duct.
- *Spleen* – this left upper quadrant solid structure is held in position by the gastrosplenic and splenorenal ligaments. It is supplied by the splenic artery (coeliac trunk) and drained by the splenic vein.
- *Adrenal glands* – appear on CT as inverted V- or Y-shaped structures are located superomedially to the kidneys. They are supplied by the superior, middle and inferior suprarenal arteries.
- *Pancreas* – this four-part (head, body, tail, uncinate process) retroperitoneal structure has its head lying to the right of the midline, within the curve of the duodenal loop, and tail pointing towards the splenic hilum. It is supplied by the superior pancreaticoduodenal artery (branch of gastroduodenal artery) and inferior pancreaticoduodenal artery (branch of superior mesenteric artery). The common bile duct descends through the head to join the pancreatic duct in forming the ampulla of Vater, which empties into the second part of the duodenum.
- *Kidneys* – these solid retroperitoneal structures (at T12–L3 level) are three to four vertebral bodies long. The right kidney lies slightly lower than the left. They are enclosed in a fibrous layer (Gerota's fascia), dividing the surrounding adipose into perinephric (inner) and paranephric (outer) fat. The renal pelvis drains anteromedially into the ureter. The kidneys are supplied by the renal arteries (right renal artery passes posterior to the IVC) and drainage is by the renal veins.
- *Ureters* – these long narrow retroperitoneal tubes descend from the renal pelvis, crossing anterior to the common iliac arteries (posterior to uterine arteries in females), and enter the pelvic brim at the level of the common iliac artery bifurcation before entering the bladder posteriorly.
- *Urinary bladder* – this low-density muscular-walled distensible structure lies above the prostate between the rectum and pubic symphysis in males, and anterior to the vagina and uterus in females.
- *Aorta* – this tubular structure pierces the diaphragm at T12 and has a retroperitoneal descent anterior to the vertebral bodies until it bifurcates into the common iliac arteries at L4.
- *IVC* – this tubular structure has a retroperitoneal ascent, lying to the right of the aorta until it pierces the diaphragm at T8.
- *Portal vein* – this tubular structure formed from the confluence of the superior mesenteric, inferior mesenteric and splenic veins runs in the hepaticoduodenal ligament with the hepatic artery and common bile duct to the porta hepatis.
- *Coeliac trunk* – the first major abdominal aortic branch subdivides into the common hepatic artery (supplies liver via proper hepatic artery, stomach and duodenum via gastroduodenal and right gastric arteries), splenic artery (supplies stomach via gastro-omental artery and spleen) and left gastric artery.
- *Superior mesenteric artery* – the second major abdominal aortic branch runs between the pancreatic head and uncinate process. Its branches supply the pancreatic head and duodenum (pancreaticoduodenal artery); ileum and jejunum (intestinal arteries); terminal ileum, caecum and appendix (ileocolic artery); ascending colon (right colic artery); proximal and mid-transverse colon (middle colic artery).
- *Inferior mesenteric artery* – the third major abdominal aortic branch supplies the distal transverse colon (left colic artery branches anastomose with middle colic artery forming the marginal artery of Drummond), descending colon (left colic artery), sigmoid colon (sigmoid branches) and upper rectum (superior rectal artery).
- *Iliac vessels* – the left and right common iliac arteries arise at the aortic bifurcation (L4) and subdivide into external and internal iliac arteries bilaterally. The external and internal iliac veins join to form the common iliac vein bilaterally. The common iliac veins ascend accompanied by their equivalent common iliac artery before merging to form the IVC at L5.

36.1 Colorectal cancer (CT with rectal contrast)

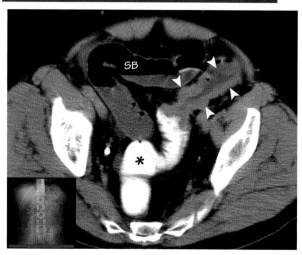

A segment of bowel wall shows circumferential irregular thickening (arrowheads). Rectal contrast material (*) introduced via a rectal catheter could not pass beyond the lesion which has obstructed the bowel. Proximal to the lesion there is dilatation of both large and small bowel (SB)

36.2 Perforation (lung windows)

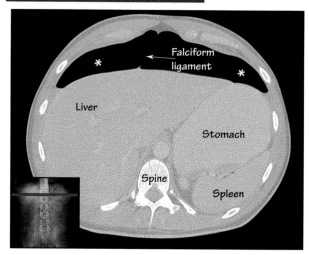

Lung window settings are highly sensitive for the presence of free intra-abdominal gas. This patient suffered an injury to the bowel from a high-speed road accident. Air (*) is seen either side of the falciform ligament separating the liver from the anterior abdominal wall

36.3 Liver metastases (portal phase intravenous enhancement)

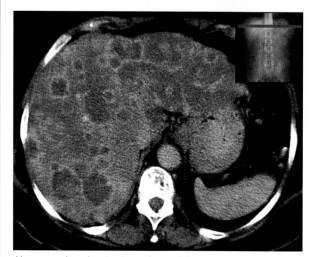

Numerous low-density irregular nodules are seen in the liver. Many of these show contrast enhancement around their rim. This patient with metastatic breast cancer had a recent ultrasound examination which had underestimated the volume of disease

36.4 Ascites

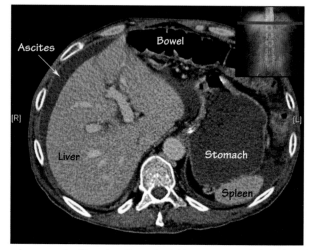

A crescent of low-density material is seen around the edge of the liver, which has a similar density to the contents of the stomach. This patient has free intra-abdominal fluid (ascites) due to peritoneal metastases from an ovarian carcinoma

Bowel pathology

- **Inflammatory bowel disease (IBD)** (see Chapter 18) – CT is useful in evaluating IBD. In Crohn's disease CT can show thickened bowel wall and intra-abdominal complications (e.g. fistulae, abscesses, small bowel obstruction). Due to the predilection for Crohn's disease to affect the small bowel, CT enteroclysis is being increasingly used to depict Crohn's disease (i.e. a volume challenge of an enteral contrast agent is administered via a nasojejunal catheter before CT imaging to distend the small bowel and improve the detection of mural abnormalities). The CT findings in ulcerative colitis are primarily thickening of the large bowel wall, which begins distally and spreads proximally in a continuous fashion.

Classic CT features of IBD

Crohn's disease
- Thickened bowel wall, often affecting terminal ileum
- Small and large bowel distribution
- Patchy inflammation
- Complications: strictures, abscesses, fistulae

Ulcerative colitis
- Thickened bowel wall
- Rectum and large bowel distribution
- Continuous inflammation
- Complications: toxic megacolon

- **Appendicitis** – this is one of the commonest causes of the acute abdomen; however, its precise aetiology remains uncertain. It may be related to occlusion by faecoliths or lymphoid hyperplasia. The inflamed appendix is distended and thick-walled and may be surrounded with periappendiceal inflammation in the surrounding fat.

Classic CT features of appendicitis

- Distended, thick-walled blind-ending tubular structure extending from the caecum
- Appendicolith
- Periappendiceal inflammation and/or fluid collection

- **Colorectal cancer** (see Chapter 28) – this is the second most common cause of cancer-related death in the developed world. The diagnosis is usually made on colonoscopy or double contrast barium enema, however, management is usually dependent on preoperative CT staging. This provides information regarding local spread, lymph node involvement and distant metastases, treatment planning including surgery and radiotherapy, and postoperative follow-up for detection of recurrence. The typical CT features of colorectal cancer are of a focal soft tissue mass or colonic wall thickening, which causes narrowing of the lumen. Local spread into the pericolic fat may be seen with loss of fat planes between the colon and adjacent organs. Any complicating features such as bowel obstruction, perforation and fistula formation may also be identified. The common sites for metastases include the liver, lungs, adrenal glands and bones and these areas are routinely imaged as part of the staging process. MRI is increasingly used to evaluate surgical resectability of rectal cancers due to its high spatial resolution in determining the relationship of the cancer with the mesorectal fascia, which is the circumferential resection margin.

Classic CT features of colorectal cancer

- Focal soft tissue colonic mass causing luminal narrowing
- Pericolic fat infiltration
- Lymph node involvement
- Complications: bowel obstruction, perforation, fistulae
- Metastases: liver, lungs, adrenal glands, bones

- **Bowel perforation** (see Chapter 17) – CT is the gold standard for detecting even tiny volumes of free gas in the abdominal cavity. Pneumoperitoneum secondary to bowel perforation is usually seen as free gas located anteriorly in the abdomen when the patient lies supine. Extraluminal gas may also be seen in pelvic abscesses of GI origin or within the adjacent mesentery in perforation secondary to diverticular disease. Gas within the bowel wall should raise the suspicion of bowel ischaemia.

Classic CT feature of bowel perforation

- Extraluminal gas (located anteriorly in supine position)

Liver lesions

Common liver lesions include benign cysts, haemangioma, cirrhosis and metastases. Primary liver malignancy is less common. Liver lesions may be detected by CT, especially in the portal venous phase of enhancement, but they are often better evaluated with US. Focal liver lesions should be localised to their appropriate segment to aid surgical planning. Each segment has its own vascular supply and biliary drainage and so may be resected independently.

Classic CT features of liver lesions

- *Cyst:* well-defined round water-dense lesion
- *Haemangioma:* well-defined lesion with peripheral enhancement that continues to enhance centripetally on delayed scans (on IV contrast imaging)
- *Cirrhosis:* shrunken, lobulated, fibrotic liver
- *Metastases:* low-density focal areas

Ascites

The causes of free fluid accumulation in the abdomen include cirrhosis, congestive heart failure, pancreatitis, peritoneal dialysis and peritoneal malignancy. Ascites is seen as water-density material in the greater and lesser sacs.

Intra-abdominal abscess

An intra-abdominal abscess is a focal collection of pus in the abdomen. These collections may develop following any infectious abdominal condition (e.g. appendicitis, diverticulitis, perforated ulcer, abdominal surgery). Aspiration and drainage of intra-abdominal collections under CT guidance is common practice, although US may also be used.

Classic CT features of abscess

- Gas/fluid level
- Gas bubbles
- Septations
- Irregular margins
- May fistulate

37.1 Pancreatic cancer

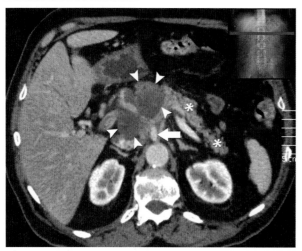

A lobulated low-density mass is seen in the head of the pancreas (arrowheads). Normal contrast enhancement of the body and tail of the pancreas is demonstrated (*). The mass has engulfed the superior mesenteric vessels (arrow) making it unresectable

37.2 Splenic trauma

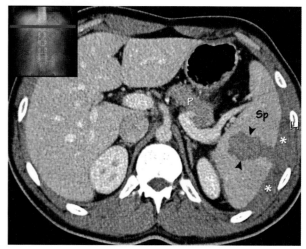

This patient had been in a road traffic accident and sustained blunt injury to the left side of the abdomen and chest. Here there is a large splenic laceration (arrowheads) with a contained splenic capsular haematoma (*). The patient was haemodynamically stable and no active extravasation of contrast is seen. Sp spleen, P pancreas

37.3 Renal cell carcinoma

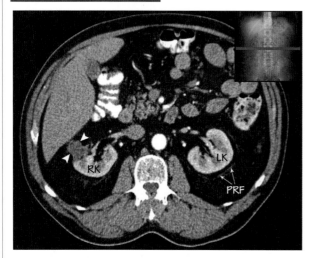

A small irregular low-density soft tissue mass (arrowheads) is arising from the lateral edge of the right kidney (RK). Despite its small size there has been breach of the perirenal fascia and the mass approaches the liver. Compare this with the left kidney (LK) and the left-sided well-defined perirenal fascia (PRF)

37.4 Abdominal aortic aneurysm

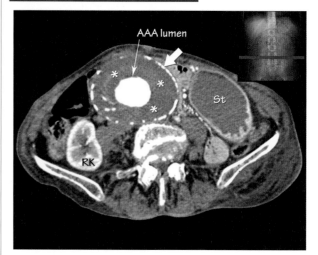

There is a very large abdominal aortic aneurysm (AAA). The outer wall is calcified (arrow) and within this there is a thick wall of soft tissue density thrombus (*). Contrast is seen flowing through the central lumen. St stomach, RK right kidney

Pancreatic lesions

• Acute pancreatitis

This is a common condition in the UK, frequently related to alcohol abuse or gallstones. Other causes of acute pancreatitis include trauma, infection, drugs and systemic diseases. The insult to the pancreas causes activation of intracellular pancreatic enzymes, which leads to autodigestion of the fatty pancreas and local vasculitis resulting in pancreatic tissue ischaemia. The severity of acute pancreatitis ranges from a mild inflammatory self-limiting reversible episode to a necrotic, septic and potentially life-threatening episode. Acute pancreatitis is often complicated by peripancreatic collections that usually develop within the first two weeks. The evaluation of the degree of necrosis by CT is important in assessing prognosis, since most life-threatening complications occur in patients with necrotising pancreatitis. The management of acute pancreatitis is supportive and CT imaging is usually delayed until at least day 4 of the acute attack when necrosis may begin to be seen. US however is performed within 24 hours of an acute attack to assess whether the aetiology is related to gallstones, which may require urgent endoscopic sphincterotomy. Acute pancreatitis can be graded in severity by CT appearances of the pancreas and surrounding tissues, and extent of pancreatic necrosis. This is called the CT Severity Index (CTSI) and provides a good indicator of prognosis.

Classic CT features of acute pancreatitis

- May be normal
- Mild pancreatic swelling due to oedema (early stages)
- Poorly enhancing areas in pancreatic parenchyma post IV contrast agent suggests ischaemia or necrosis
- Complications: infected necrotic pancreas (gas within pancreas), extrapancreatic fluid collections, pseudocyst, venous thrombosis

---

• Pancreatic cancer

Most pancreatic cancers are adenocarcinomas with a poor prognosis. The presentation is variable (e.g. pancreatic head tumours present with weight loss and obstructive jaundice whereas tumours of the pancreatic body and tail usually present with pain and weight loss). CT is useful in diagnosis, biopsy, staging and management planning (e.g. determining the feasibility of resection). The CT appearances of pancreatic adenocarcinoma are also variable. They may be low, high or isodense soft tissue masses, which are hypo-or hypervascular and may cause biliary and pancreatic duct obstruction with proximal dilatation. CT-guided biopsy is often therefore required to obtain a histological diagnosis.

Classic CT features of pancreatic cancer

- Hypodense/isodense/hyperdense soft tissue mass
- Hypo/hypervascular
- May cause biliary and pancreatic duct dilatation

Splenic lesions

Blunt splenic trauma is the commonest indication for imaging the spleen with CT. It can identify and quantify splenic injury by detecting intravenous contrast agent extravasation, often called 'contrast blush'. CT is also useful in following the progress of splenic injuries in conservatively managed patients.

Classic CT features of splenic trauma

- Perisplenic intravenous contrast agent extravasation (contrast blush)
- Splenic laceration

Kidney and adrenal gland lesions

The commonest kidney lesions include cysts, calculi and tumours. Simple renal cysts are completely benign and well-defined water-dense lesions on CT. Cysts that have more complex architecture (e.g. irregular border, septations, calcification) raise the suspicion for malignancy (e.g. renal cell carcinoma). Lesions that are irregular, solid, disturb the renal contour, and enhance with IV contrast agent are likely to be malignant. Renal cell carcinoma commonly metastasises to the lungs and bone.

Adenomas are the commonest adrenal lesion. These are benign and appear as a small soft tissue mass in one of the limbs of the gland. The second most common adrenal lesion is metastatic cancer, which appears as a soft tissue mass of varying size arising from the gland. Cancers that metastasise to the adrenal glands include lung, breast, melanoma, kidney, thyroid and colon cancer.

Classic CT features of kidney lesions

• **Cyst**	Well-defined, water-dense lesion
• **Malignancy**	Irregular, enhancing solid soft tissue mass

Classic CT features of adrenal lesions

• **Adenoma**	Small fat-dense lesion
• **Metastases**	Soft tissue mass (varying size)

Abdominal aortic aneurysm (AAA)

AAA is an abnormal focal dilatation of the abdominal aorta, which is 50% greater than the normal aortic diameter. The normal infrarenal aortic diameter is 2 cm and so AAA is present if the diameter is 3 cm or more. The risk of rupture is low until the aneurysm reaches 5.5 cm, when open surgical or endovascular repair is usually indicated. Rapidly expanding aneurysms (>1 cm/year) are also at high risk of rupture and require urgent repair. When IV contrast agent is used, CT imaging allows measurement of the absolute size of the aneurysm and the presence of mural thrombus and dissection. CT is also used for follow up of endovascular graft repairs.

Classic CT features of AAA

- Infrarenal aortic diameter 3 cm or more
- Mural thrombus
- Calcification

38.1 Axial CT brain: normal

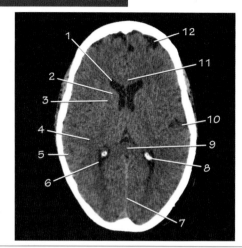

38.2 Axial CT brain: normal

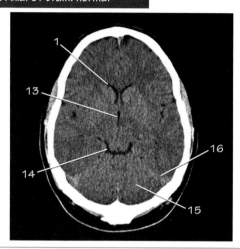

38.3 Axial CT brain: normal

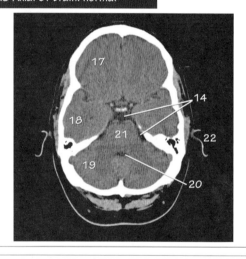

Key

1 Lateral ventricle (anterior horn)	19 Posterior cranial fossa
2 Caudate nucleus	20 Fourth ventricle
3 Internal capsule	21 Pons
4 White matter	22 Pinna of ear
5 Grey matter	23 Frontal air sinuses
6 Lateral ventricle (posterior horn)	24 Orbit
7 Falx cerebri	25 Cochlea within petrous
8 Choroid plexus (calcified)	temporal bone
9 Corpus callosum (splenium)	26 External auditory meatus
10 Sylvian fissure	27 Jugular foramen
11 Corpus callosum (genu)	28 Occipital bone
12 Sulci	29 Mastoid air cells
13 Third ventricle	30 Squamous temporal bone
14 Basal cisterns	31 Greater wing of the sphenoid
15 Cerebellum	32 Frontal bone
16 Tentorium cerebelli	33 Ethmoid air cells
17 Anterior cranial fossa	34 Sphenoid sinus
18 Middle cranial fossa	35 Semicircular canal
	36 Internal auditory meatus

38.4 Axial CT skull base: normal

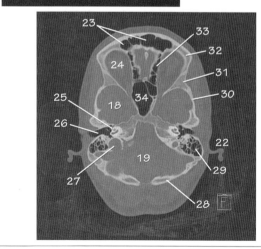

38.5 Axial CT skull base: normal

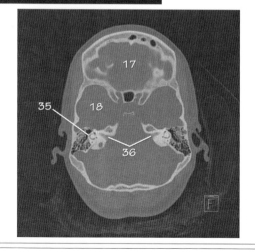

CT is the primary modality for imaging the brain. A scout view is usually acquired in the sagittal plane before thin and thick transverse/axial sections are acquired parallel to the skull base. The data can then be used to construct sagittal and coronal images.

Extracranial structures

• *Subcutaneous fat* – this is seen as a rim of low-density soft tissue surrounding the skull.
• *Muscles* – these are seen as smooth mid-density structures inserting into and arising from bone (e.g. the muscles of mastication).
• *Pinna* – the soft tissue structure of the external ear.
• *Temporal arteries* – these may be visible as tubular structures, anterior to the external auditory meatus.
• *Orbital structures* – the globe of the eye, optic nerve and extraocular muscles may be seen on the inferior slices of the CT imaging series.

Cranium

• *Frontal bone* – this forms the forehead, and the roof of each orbit and nasal cavity.
• *Parietal bones (paired)* – these form the skull roof.
• *Temporal bones (paired)* – these contribute to the lateral walls of the skull, and to the skull base where they house the auditory apparatus.
• *Occipital bone* – this forms the posterior skull wall and contributes to the skull base. It contains the foramen magnum, which allows passage of the spinal cord from the cranium to the spinal canal.
• *Sphenoid bone* – this contributes to the skull base, where it forms the sella turcica to accommodate the pituitary gland. It also forms the optic canals for passage of the optic nerves from each orbit to the brain. The sphenoid also forms the posterior part of the orbital wall.
• *Ethmoid bone* – this contributes to the skull base, roof of the nasal cavity, and walls of the orbit.
• *Skull base* – this is divided into the anterior cranial fossa (frontal and ethmoid bones), middle cranial fossa (temporal and sphenoid bones) and posterior cranial fossa (occipital bone). The skull base contains multiple foramina for the passage of cranial nerves and vessels.
• *Air spaces* – there are four sets of paranasal sinuses, which are air-filled bony spaces that communicate with the nasal cavity (sphenoid, ethmoid, frontal and maxillary). Mastoid air cells are tiny air-filled spaces within the mastoid process of the temporal bone.

Intracranial structures

• *Cerebrum* – this is the part of the brain lying above the tentorium cerebelli, a fibrous sheet of dura mater, separating it from the cerebellum. The cerebrum is divided into structurally (but not physiologically) symmetrical hemispheres by the falx cerebri, another sheet of dura mater which passes in the sagittal midline. Each hemisphere has four lobes: frontal, temporal, parietal and occipital. The hemispheres are composed of grey (cortical) and white (subcortical) matter arranged in gyral folds, separated by sulci. Grey matter (neuronal cell bodies and glial cells) has a higher soft tissue density compared with white matter (myelinated axonal tracts) and therefore appears brighter on CT. The basal ganglia are a group of nuclei (putamen, caudate nucleus, globus pallidus, subthalamic nucleus and substantia nigra) located within each hemisphere and involved with cognition, motor control, emotions and learning. The internal capsule is an area of white matter containing axons that connect the cerebral cortex above to the brainstem and spinal cord below.
• *Cerebellum* – this is the part of the brain that occupies the posterior fossa and lies beneath the tentorium cerebelli. The cerebellum influences coordination, sensory perception and motor control. The cerebellar peduncles are stalk-like masses of nerve fibres connecting the cerebellar cortex to the brainstem and other components of the central nervous system.
• *Brainstem* – this is divided into the midbrain, pons and medulla. It passes through the foramen magnum in the skull base to become the spinal cord.
• *Meninges* – these are a protective coating surrounding the brain and spinal cord and are comprised of three layers. The outer layer (dura mater) is thick and fibrous and is in contact with the skull. The middle layer (arachnoid mater) is thin and fibrous with spider-like projections attaching it to the inner layer. The inner layer (pia mater) is a thin delicate membrane, tightly wrapped around the surface of the brain and spinal cord. The space between the arachnoid mater and pia mater (subarachnoid space) is filled with cerebrospinal fluid (CSF) and contains blood vessels.
• *Ventricular system* – this is responsible for CSF circulation produced by its choroid plexus. It is comprised of four ventricles connected by small channels and apertures through which CSF may flow. The right and left lateral ventricles are connected via the foramina of Monroe to the third ventricle, which is connected to the fourth ventricle by the Sylvian aqueduct. CSF exits the fourth ventricle through the central canal of the spinal cord and through other apertures to flow into the cisterns of the subarachnoid space. CSF then flows over the cerebral hemispheres and around the spinal cord within the spinal canal.
• *Pituitary and pineal gland* – the pituitary gland is a soft tissue structure sitting in the sella turcica of the sphenoid bone. The pineal gland may calcify and is therefore seen as a high-density structure posterior to the third ventricle in the midline.
• *Vessels* – the internal carotid and basilar arteries can be seen entering the skull and anastamosing at the circle of Willis (located in the centre of axial slices at the level of the sella turcica). Cerebral veins drain to the venous sinuses, which are contained within the dura mater. The largest of these sinuses is the superior sagittal sinus (superior midline), which drains into the transverse and sigmoid sinuses (located laterally along the inside of the occipital bone), which then drain into the internal jugular vein.

39.1 Extradural haemorrhage (EDH): axial CT

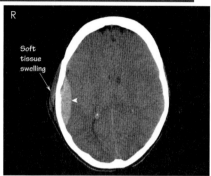

A lens-shaped area of high density is seen within the skull on the right (arrowhead). This is the typical appearance of an extradural haemorrhage which usually arises following injury to the middle meningeal artery. There was an underlying fracture of the temporal bone in this patient seen on bone window settings

39.2 Subdural haematoma (SDH): axial CT

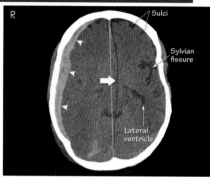

A crescentic rim of high-density material (acute blood) is seen over the surface of the right cerebral hemisphere (arrowheads). There is evidence of mass effect with effacement of the sulci, Sylvian fissure, and lateral ventricle (compare with left), with shift of midline structures (green to red line)

39.3 Subarachnoid haemorrhage (SAH): axial CT

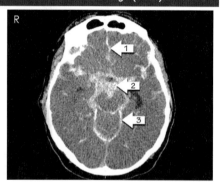

There is widespread high-density material (acute blood) within the subarachnoid space. The blood is seen in the interhemispheric fissure (1), the suprasellar cistern (2), and is layered over the tentorium cerebelli (3). The underlying cause was an aneurysm found on CT angiography

39.4 Intracerebral haemorrhage (ICH): axial CT

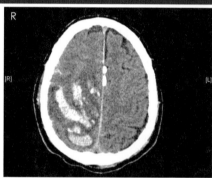

Areas of high density represent acute intracerebral haemorrhage of the right cerebral hemisphere. The high-density areas (blood) are surrounded by low-density areas (oedema). Mass effect is seen with loss of sulci on this side and slight midline shift

39.5 Cerebral infarction: axial CT

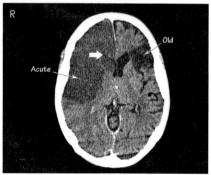

On the right there is a large low-density area indicating an acute infarction of the right middle cerebral artery (MCA) territory. This is causing mass effect with loss of sulci, effacement of the right lateral ventricle anterior horn (arrow) and some midline shift. For comparison an old low density infarct is seen on the left

39.6 Cerebral tumour: axial CT post-contrast

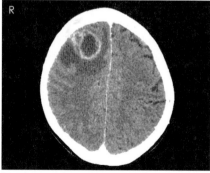

A peripherally enhancing lesion is seen in the right cerebral hemisphere. Note its central low-density area (necrosis) and the surrounding low density (oedema). Mass effect is seen with sulcal effacement on this side and slight deviation of the falx cerebri. Biopsy proved this to be a malignant tumour

Intracranial haemorrhage

A head CT is performed without an intravenous contrast agent to detect acute bleeding. This is because blood is dense and therefore difficult to distinguish from intravenous contrast agent. The appearance of a haemorrhage on CT imaging changes with time, and so correlation with the onset of clinical symptoms and signs is essential. Acute blood is bright but becomes darker over the next few days. After one month a haematoma becomes the same density as CSF.

Extradural haematoma (EDH)

EDH is a collection of blood between the skull and dura mater. It is most often due to arterial bleeding following head trauma. The majority are located in the temporoparietal region and caused by bleeding from the middle meningeal artery secondary to a skull fracture, which is present in up to 90% of cases. CT imaging features of acute EDH include:

• Well-demarcated 'lentiform' (biconvex) high density extra-axial (outside the brain) collection.
• Rarely crosses suture lines between cranial bones because dura mater is firmly attached to the skull at sutures.
• Air within EDH suggests an open fracture, or a fracture of the paranasal sinuses or mastoid air cells.

Subdural haematoma (SDH)

SDH is a collection of extra-axial blood between the dura mater and arachnoid mater. It is most often due to venous bleeding from bridging veins that traverse the subdural space following head trauma and deceleration injuries. It may also be seen in shaken baby syndrome, patients with coagulopathy, and in cerebral atrophy (where minimal trauma can cause significant bleeding due to increased tension on the bridging veins). SDH may lead to raised intracranial pressure and cause displacement of midline structures to the contralateral side. CT imaging features of acute SDH include:

• 'Crescentic' high density extra-axial collection conforming to the cerebral convexity (although can become lentiform).
• Crosses suture lines as collection is subdural.
• Moderate and large SDH can cause midline shift.
• Falx cerebri appears dense, thickened and irregular with interhemispheric SDH (associated with non-accidental injury in children).

Subarachnoid haemorrhage (SAH)

SAH is bleeding into the subarachnoid space (space between the arachnoid mater and pia mater which contains CSF). It most often occurs spontaneously from a ruptured aneurysm in the circle of Willis and patients typically complain of sudden-onset extreme severe headache. CT imaging typically reveals high-density blood in the CSF spaces (ventricular system, over cerebral hemispheres, Sylvian fissure, basal cisterns). If SAH is confirmed, a CT angiogram or a conventional cerebral angiogram is performed. If CT imaging is negative but the clinical suspicion is high and there are no contraindications, lumbar puncture should be performed for detection of xanthochromia.

Intracerebral haemorrhage (ICH)

ICH is bleeding into the brain parenchyma (intra-axial). It is also known as haemorrhagic stroke and is the second most common cause of a cerebrovascular event after ischaemic stroke. CT imaging allows differentiation of a haemorrhagic event from an ischaemic event, which dictates subsequent management of these conditions. The greatest risk factors are hypertension and anticoagulation therapy. Other causes include penetrating trauma, deceleration injuries, rupture of an intracerebral aneurysm, or bleeding from an arteriovenous malformation or tumour. Patients usually present with neurological deficit.

Cerebral infarction

Cerebral infarction is caused by a sudden perfusion deficit to an area of the brain resulting in corresponding loss of neurological function. This is known as ischaemic stroke, which is the commonest cause of a cerebrovascular event. If the neurological deficit lasts less than 24 hours the event is termed a transient ischaemic attack (TIA). Thromboembolic events are by far the commonest cause. Thrombosis most often occurs at cerebral artery branch points and is related to vascular wall damage and hypercoagulable states. Emboli may arise from atherosclerotic plaques of extracranial arteries or thrombus originating from the heart. CT imaging features of cerebral infarction evolve over time. Within the first three hours of symptom onset, a faint low-density area may be seen affecting a vascular territory of the brain parenchyma. Between 6 and 12 hours, there is usually sufficient cell swelling (cytotoxic oedema) to produce a CT-identifiable region of low density affecting both the grey and white matter. Subsequent bleeding into the area of infarction may occur from the damaged blood vessels, which causes high density within the low-density infarct. Infarction is often accompanied by oedema, which may cause a mass effect ranging from minor sulcal effacement to shift of midline structures. In the following weeks to months, the infarct is resorbed by macrophages, leaving it appearing as an area of low density (dark) affecting both grey and white matter.

Intracranial tumours

Intracranial tumours may be primary or metastatic. Most are solitary primary tumours arising from brain parenchyma or other related tissues (vessels, nerves, meninges, pituitary, lymphatics, skull). Metastatic tumours are often multiple and typically from cancers such as lung, breast, melanoma, and renal cancers. The clinical presentation of brain tumours varies with their site and size but includes headaches, seizures, focal neurological deficits and signs of raised intracranial pressure (e.g. papilloedema). CT imaging is initially performed without a contrast agent and then with a contrast agent if a space-occupying lesion (SOL) is suspected radiologically or clinically. Brain tumours usually cause disruption of the blood–brain barrier resulting in vasogenic oedema from capillary leakage, which spares the grey matter. Most tumours enhance on contrast agent CT imaging and are often surrounded by a halo of low-density subcortical oedema with varying degrees of mass effect.

Classic CT head features

• **Haemorrhage**	High density (acute), density drops over few days, CSF density after 1 month (chronic)
• **EDH**	'Lentiform', rarely crosses sutures, usually associated with skull fracture
• **SDH**	'Crescentic', usually crosses sutures
• **SAH**	Blood in CSF spaces, e.g. ventricles
• **ICH**	Intra-axial/parenchymal blood
• **Infarct**	Low density in vascular territory, grey and white matter affected, cytotoxic oedema
• **Tumour**	Typically enhancing focal parenchymal lesion, vasogenic oedema

40.1 KUB control image

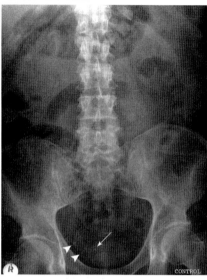

There are several small densities projected over the right side of the pelvis. Subsequent IVU images showed that two of these (arrowheads) were phleboliths (venous calcification) but there was also a vesico-ureteric junction (VUJ) calculus/stone (arrow)

40.2 '10 minute' image

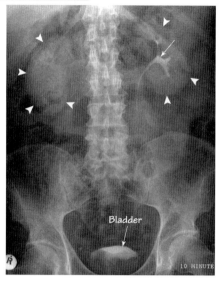

There is uptake of contrast by the renal parenchyma bilaterally forming an outline of both kidneys (arrowheads). On the left there is normal excretion of contrast into the renal collecting system (arrow). Contrast is also seen collecting in the bladder

40.3 Post micturition image

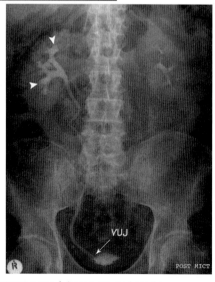

A '20 minute image' demonstrated similar appearances with 'clubbed' or dilated calyces (arrowheads) and a column of contrast agent. Post-micturition this column persisted with the ureter filling from the VUJ upwards. The level of obstruction is identical to the position of the VUJ stone on the control image (see fig 40.1)

40.4 CT KUB

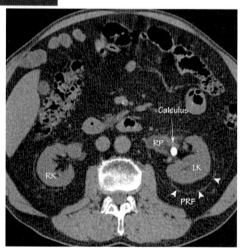

This patient had a history of recurrent renal colic due to renal calculi. Here a calculus is seen in the renal pelvis (RP) of the left kidney (LK). RK right kidney, PRF perirenal fascia

Intravenous urogram (IVU)

An IVU is a contrast agent enhanced radiological study of the urinary tract allowing anomalies of the kidneys, ureters and bladder to be identified. It is most commonly performed in patients who present with renal colic (with or without microscopic haematuria) to search for renal calculi and obstruction. IVU may also reveal other renal abnormalities including renal cell carcinoma and congenital variants (horseshoe kidney, duplex kidney, ureteric duplication). A pre-contrast agent plain X-ray of the kidneys, ureters and bladder (KUB) is taken at the start to serve as a 'control' for identifying any radio-opaque calculi in the urinary tract and other possible causes for the patient's symptoms (e.g. gallstones, bowel obstruction, aortic aneurysm). The IV contrast agent is administered via a peripheral vein (approximately 1 ml/kg body weight) if the patient's renal function is adequate and there is no history of adverse reaction (see Chapter 6). The contrast agent is subsequently filtered by the kidneys and concentrated in the urinary tract where it is visible on X-ray imaging. X-ray images including the kidneys, ureters and bladder are taken at set time intervals in order to delineate the anatomy and identify any pathology as the contrast agent passes through the urinary system.

In the absence of obstruction, a nephrogram (opacification of the renal parenchyma by contrast agent in the renal tubules appearing as a kidney-shaped opacity) is visible in less than a minute, which signifies the contrast agent has reached the renal cortex. At approximately 5 minutes post contrast agent injection, the renal calyces and pelvis opacify. The next film is usually taken at approximately 15 minutes post contrast agent injection to demonstrate opacification within the ureters and possibly the bladder. Finally, an image is acquired post micturition to confirm free drainage of the contrast agent from the urinary system and to exclude any bladder pathology. In the presence of delayed excretion of the contrast agent, further images are acquired at later intervals until the contrast agent dissipates. This provides information to assess the degree of obstruction and plan further management (e.g. nephrostomy, percutaneous nephrolithotomy, ureteric stent). The complete image series is then evaluated to interpret the following.

1 *Kidneys* – symmetry, size, position, outline, contrast uptake and excretion.

2 *Ureters* – symmetry, size, calibre (a normal ureter is not usually fully visible on a single image due to peristalsis), smoothness, presence of a 'standing column' (continuous column of ureteric opacification from the kidney to a distal cut-off point with no opacification beyond suggests an obstruction at this point).

3 *Bladder* – size, shape, outline, and voiding (post micturition).

A dilated tract is usually a sign of chronic obstruction whereas acute obstruction causes a dense nephrogram with or without a standing column.

Urinary tract calculi

Urinary tract calculi or stones are largely composed of oxalate (pure oxalate, calcium oxalate), uric acid, or cystine. Not all stones are visible on KUB because they may be small or radiolucent (uric acid stones), or due to overlying stool or bone. In addition, numerous other calcifications may mimic the appearance of urinary stones, e.g. vascular calcifications, phleboliths (lucent centres), appendicoliths, calcified masses and bowel contents (including retained barium contrast). Predisposing factors for urinary stone formation include urinary stasis (e.g. structural abnormality, obstruction), metabolic anomalies (e.g. hyperparathyroidism, hypercalcaemia, hypercalciuria, cystinuria) and infection (e.g. *Proteus mirabilis*). Calculi mostly form in the renal calyces but can migrate anywhere along the urinary tract. The usual presentation is acute renal colic (sudden onset pain in the flank radiating towards the groin) with associated microscopic haematuria, nausea and vomiting. On examination the patient is typically restless and often has costovertebral angle tenderness. Urinary tract sepsis in the presence of an obstructed system is an emergency and requires immediate intervention, commonly by percutaneous nephrostomy. The clinical course of urinary stones is variable, but in general, the smaller the stone the more likely it is to pass spontaneously (90% pass if <4 mm, 50% pass if <7 mm, unlikely to pass without intervention if >7 mm). Large pelvicalyceal and staghorn calculi usually require intervention.

Classic IVU features of urinary calculi

• **Plain kidneys/ureters/ bladder X-ray (KUB)**	Radio-opaque bodies along urinary tract
• **Post contrast agent images**	
	Filling defects within opacified tract
	Delay in contrast excretion with dense persistent nephrogram
	Tract dilatation +/– enlarged pelvicalyceal system
	Standing column post micturition

CT KUB (kidneys/ureters/bladder)

In many centres, CT KUB has replaced IVU as the primary imaging modality for urinary tract disorders. A non-contrast agent enhanced CT KUB with thin slices is the most sensitive method of imaging for detecting urinary tract stones; however, radiolucent stones are not readily visible. A contrast agent is not used as it opacifies the entire urinary tract and may mask the presence of stones. A contrast agent enhanced study may be subsequently performed if there are unexpected findings. Plain X-ray imaging also has a role to visualise the size, shape and position of urinary stones with follow-up studies to monitor movement of the stones and confirm complete excretion from the body. The advantages of CT KUB include its ability to reveal alternative pathology which may mimic the symptoms of an obstructed urinary tract (e.g. appendicitis, UTI, diverticulitis, ovarian pathology) or other incidental findings (e.g. abdominal aortic aneurysm). CT KUB can be performed rapidly and avoids the use of an intravenous contrast agent, which may be contraindicated in some patients (see Chapter 6). The drawbacks of CT KUB include the high initial radiation dose, the absence of individual renal function assessment, and its unsuitability for monitoring the passage of stones.

41.1 CT Pulmonary angiogram: pulmonary embolus

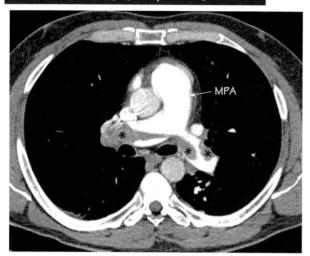

This patient presented with shortness of breath and chest pain 10 days after a gynaecological operation. The main pulmonary artery (MPA) is dilated and within the right and left pulmonary arteries there are filling defects (*) of soft tissue density due to a large pulmonary embolus. This crosses the midline forming a 'saddle'

41.2 CT Aorta angiogram: aortic dissection

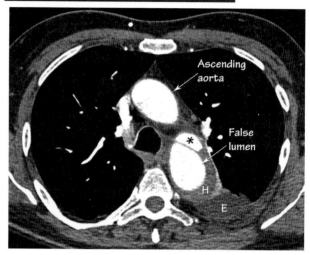

There is a large 'false lumen' of the descending aorta. This arises distal to the left subclavian artery (not shown). The 'true lumen' (*) remains patent but it is compressed by the false lumen. Other features that often accompany aortic dissections are the unopacified mural/wall haematoma (H) and a left-sided pleural effusion (E). This patient presented with tearing interscapular pain typical of an aortic dissection

41.3 Renal MR angiogram: renal artery stenosis

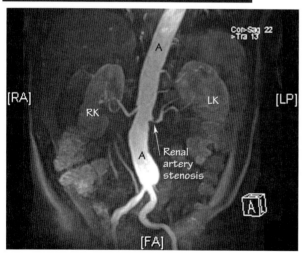

MR angiography of this patient with hypertension revealed a stenosis at the origin of the left renal artery. This type of lesion is often treated radiologically with balloon dilatation or stent insertion under imaging guidance. A aorta, LK left kidney, RK right kidney

41.4 Cerebral CT angiogram: cerebral aneurysm

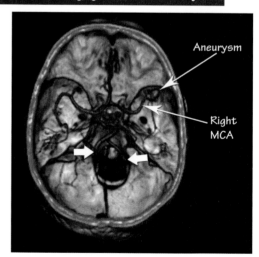

This patient presented with a subarachnoid haemorrhage. For a CT angiogram contrast agent is administered intravenously and tracked to the carotid arteries. Images are acquired as the contrast agent passes through the cerebral arteries. The brain tissue is then 'removed' using imaging software. There is a right middle cerebral artery (MCA) aneurysm which was treated by embolisation under imaging guidance. The entire cerebral circulation is shown including the vertebral arteries (arrows)

CT angiography (CTA)

CTA is an excellent imaging investigation to evaluate the vascular system. It uses IV contrast agent, which is administered peripherally, and then operates a 'bolus tracking' CT technique. This entails tracking the contrast agent bolus until it reaches the region of interest. At this point the CT scanner is triggered to follow the bolus through the region of interest and acquire optimally enhanced images throughout. The drawbacks of CTA include the radiation exposure and the adverse risks of iodinated contrast agents, including CIN (see Chapter 6), which can pose a conundrum in patients with pre-existing poor renal function.

MR angiography (MRA)

MRA is an excellent investigation to evaluate the vascular system. The scanning time is longer than CTA but it may be performed with or without a contrast agent and does not use ionising radiation. However, patients with implanted pacemakers and defibrillators, cochlear implants and brain aneurysm clips cannot be scanned by MR. There is also a small risk of NSF with the use of gadolinium (see Chapter 6).

Common applications of CTA and MRA

• *Coronary artery disease* – assessing the distribution and extent of coronary artery disease prior to intervention (e.g. angioplasty, stenting, coronary artery bypass grafting).

• *Carotid artery disease* – assessing atherosclerotic disease in the carotid arteries in patients at risk of stroke.

• *Renal artery disease* – assessing renal blood flow in patients with renal artery stenosis and in assessing suitability for renal transplantation.

• *Peripheral vascular disease* – assessing peripheral vascular disease in the limbs to plan surgical repair (e.g. bypass grafting) or endovascular repair (e.g. angioplasty and stenting). CTA is also used for follow-up post repair.

• *Pulmonary embolism* – detecting emboli in the pulmonary arterial tree. This is known as CT pulmonary angiography (CTPA).

• *Aneurysm* – identifying and evaluating aneurysms of the aorta and most other important vessels, including those in the brain.

• *Arteriovenous malformation* – identifying and evaluating arteriovenous malformations, which often occur in the brain.

• *Vascular trauma* – identifying and assessing vascular injury in trauma patients.

• *Dissection* – identifying and evaluating aortic dissection and other major vessels.

• *Cancer* – evaluating a tumour's vascular supply is important prior to intervention (e.g. surgery, chemoembolisation, selective internal radiotherapy).

42.1 MRI referral checklist

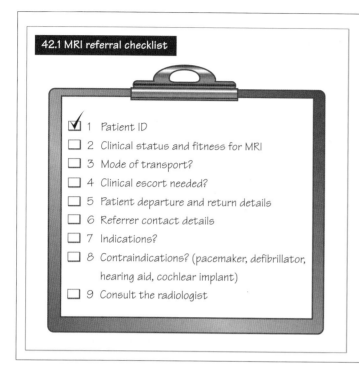

1 Patient ID
2 Clinical status and fitness for MRI
3 Mode of transport?
4 Clinical escort needed?
5 Patient departure and return details
6 Referrer contact details
7 Indications?
8 Contraindications? (pacemaker, defibrillator, hearing aid, cochlear implant)
9 Consult the radiologist

42.2 Approach to MRI interpretation

1 Identify sequence
2 Identify key structures with respect to their signal intensity
3 Assess for pathology, aberrant anatomy and physiology

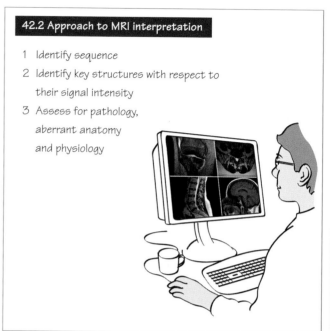

MRI referral checklist (see Chapter 7)

The referrer carries the responsibility to ensure the correct and complete information is conveyed to the Imaging Department so that the patient is appropriately diagnosed and managed.

• **Patient identification:** The referrer must ensure that the Imaging Department receives the correct identification details of the patient to be investigated: full name, date of birth and hospital identification number are the essentials.

• **Clinical status:** The referrer must convey the patient's clinical condition and urgency of the referral to the Imaging Department. MRI is rarely one of the primary investigations for most acute symptoms and signs. Occasionally, conditions such as suspected cauda equina syndrome need to be managed more urgently with MRI.

• **Patient mobility:** MRI scans can take more than an hour to complete and, in order to obtain optimal images, the patient is required to lie still for this period of time. The referrer should therefore consider the patient's condition with respect to their ability to comply with the investigation protocol. In children, MRI is often performed under general anaesthetic. Due to the strength of the magnetic field, ferrous material cannot be taken directly into the MR scanner room, which includes the cardiac defibrillator and other adjunctive resuscitation kit.

Consequently, unstable patients should only undergo MRI if absolutely necessary, with the emergency team on standby outside the MR scanner room.

• **Patient location and travel details:** The need for a clinical escort should be conveyed and the points of departure and return and contact details must also be notified to the Imaging Department to ensure the patient is transferred safely and efficiently.

• **Indications:** MRI can reveal a wide range of pathology, especially in the soft tissues, and its application is rapidly expanding. Well-established uses include imaging of the brain and spinal cord, muscles and ligaments, the heart and vascular system, and rectal cancers. The referral indication should always include a salient history and a specific question to be answered by MRI. The radiologist should be consulted in most cases.

• **Contraindications:** MRI is a safe, non-invasive investigation. However, there are a few important contraindications primarily related to the magnetic field. These include patients with a pacemaker or defibrillator devices, and hearing aids or cochlear implants. Orthopaedic internal fixation devices are usually safe after a few months. The long-term effects of strong magnetic fields on the foetus are yet unknown and so it is advisable to delay MRI in pregnant women, unless it is clinically crucial.

Approach to MRI interpretation

MRI began in the 1970s, but in the early years it was an enigma to even senior radiologists. In recent times, however, MRI has undergone huge expansion impacting on many areas of clinical medicine. This has been primarily driven by faster image acquisition times and the high level of detail seen in the images. A basic approach to understanding an MRI series begins with identifying the *image sequence* (see Chapter 5). Tissues have different signal characteristics depending on which sequence has been selected. T1- and T2-weighted sequences are amongst the most routinely used.

MRI is an excellent and useful imaging tool in the following:

- Gastrointestinal (hepatobiliary and rectal) system
- Musculoskeletal system
- Neurological system
- Cardiac system
- Vascular system
- Gynaecological system
- Oncology
- Breast disease.

Signal intensities of tissues on T1- and T2-weighted image sequences

	T1 weighted	T2 weighted
White	Fatty tissue Posterior pituitary gland Paramagnetic contrast agents (gadolinium)	High free water tissue (CSF, bladder, gall bladder) Oedema Protein tissue (abscess, synovial fluid) Fatty tissue (not as bright as T1)
Light/mid grey	Organs and soft tissue structures	Organs and soft tissue structures
Dark grey/black	Air Bone/ligaments/tendons Stones Fast-flowing blood	Air Bone/ligaments/tendons Stones Fast-flowing blood

43.1 Sagittal brain MRI : T1 (left) and T2 (right)

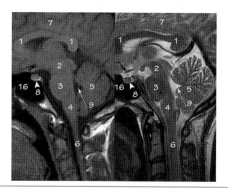

43.2 Axial brain MRI: T2 at level of lateral ventricles (left) and T2 at level of cerebellum (right)

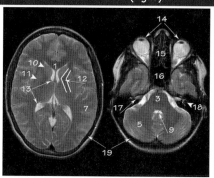

Key

1	Corpus callosum
2	Midbrain
3	Pons
4	Medulla oblongata
5	Cerebellum
6	Spinal cord
7	Cerebrum
8	Pituitary gland
9	Fourth ventricle
10	Caudate nucleus
11	Lentiform nucleus
12	Internal capsule
13	Lateral ventricle
14	Eyes
15	Ethmoid air cells
16	Sphenoid sinus
17	Internal auditory meatus
18	Cochlea
19	Skull

43.3 Multiple sclerosis: axial T2 at level above lateral ventricles

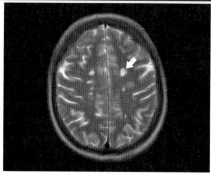

There are multiple bilateral foci of high signal (arrow) present within the white matter (appears dark on T2). These lesions lie immediately above and to the side of the lateral ventricles. The periventricular white matter is a typical location for multiple sclerosis lesions

43.4 Cerebral infarction: DWI (left) and ADC (right)

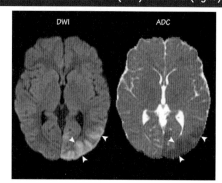

The DWI shows bright signal (arrowheads) in the distribution of the left posterior cerebral artery. The ADC image shows this area as low signal and therefore it is not due to T2 signal (note the bright ventricles). This is evidence of restricted diffusion which is a sign of infarction. DWI is the most sensitive investigation for acute cerebral infarction

43.5 Pituitary tumour: sagittal T1 images pre- and post-gadolinium injection

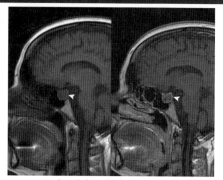

This patient presented with headaches and visual field disturbance (bitemporal hemianopia). The pre-contrast image (left) shows a pituitary adenoma (arrowhead) which demonstrates abnormal enhancement on the post-contrast scan (right). This is classified as a macroadenoma (>1 cm). The bigger a pituitary lesion becomes the more likely it is to cause visual disturbance due to compression of the optic chiasm which lies immediately above the pituitary gland

MR imaging of the head

The neuroanatomy seen on MR imaging is similar to that seen on CT imaging (see Chapter 38), however, MR imaging allows visualisation of structures with greater differentiation and detail even without the use of contrast agent enhancement. The MR imaging series of the brain are viewed in a similar format to CT images (axial, sagittal and coronal planes). MR also has the advantage of viewing the brainstem without the significant artefact limitations of CT images. The standard MR imaging investigation of the brain includes T1-weighted, T2-weighted, proton density weighted (PD) and fluid-attenuated inversion recovery sequences (FLAIR). T1-weighted images with gadolinium enhancement may also be acquired. Each of these acquisition sequences demonstrates different patterns of tissue signal characteristics, which commonly forms the basis of interpretation and diagnosis (see Chapter 42).

• *T1-weighted acquisition sequences* – the signal intensity on T1-weighted acquisitions depends on the fat content of the tissues in question. Subcutaneous fat appears very bright and the myelin sheaths of white matter appear brighter than grey matter. CSF and pathological fluid appear dark. T1-weighted images are best at defining anatomy due to their excellent spatial resolution. In the brain, however, they are also useful in conjunction with T2-weighted images to distinguish blood from other pathology, estimate the age of a haemorrhage and differentiate fatty lesions from other pathology.

• *T2-weighted acquisition sequences* – the signal intensity on T2-weighted acquisitions depends on the water content of the tissues in question. CSF is very bright and can be easily identified within the different components of the ventricular system and subarachnoid space. Fat is darker than on T1-weighted acquisitions and so white matter appears darker than grey matter. T2-weighted images are often the best sequence for evaluating pathology. This is because pathological lesions often contain water and are therefore bright and easily seen on T2. This is true for infective processes, tumours, and inflammatory conditions such as multiple sclerosis, which typically reveals bright plaques on T2-weighted images.

• *Proton density (PD) acquisition sequences* – this sequence is acquired at the same time as the T2 sequence. The signal intensity on PD-weighted acquisitions depends on the number of protons per unit tissue. Tissues with a high number of protons are bright (e.g. CSF) and those with a low number of protons are dark. PD sequences are often helpful, but pathological fluid is usually more easily differentiated from other structures on different sequences, such as FLAIR.

• *FLAIR acquisition sequences* – this is similar to T2 except the bright signal from CSF is suppressed. This allows clearer evaluation of T2-bright lesions, especially those near CSF-filled spaces (e.g. white matter plaque adjacent to the ventricular system).

Intracranial haemorrhage

Intracranial haemorrhage may be diagnosed and evaluated by MRI.

MR imaging is superior to CT imaging for detecting haemorrhage in the subacute and chronic phases. However, CT imaging remains the preferred modality in the acute setting because it is much faster.

The signal intensity of haemorrhage changes with time on both T1- and T2-weighted sequences. This is because the breakdown products of blood clots induce various artefacts. Initially, artefact is due to the presence of oxygenated haemoglobin, which is dark on T1 and bright on T2. After several hours, deoxyhaemoglobin is predominant and this is dark on both T1 and T2. After approximately three days, there is an increasing amount of intracellular methaemoglobin, which is bright on T1 but dark on T2, and then free methaemoglobin which is bright on both. Eventually, over months, methaemoglobin is exchanged for haemosiderin, which is dark on both sequences. In order to accurately direct management the timing of any haemorrhagic event should be established from the history.

Cerebral infarction and diffusion-weighted MRI (DW-MRI)

When there is a sudden perfusion deficit to the brain, the glial cells undergo ischaemic change, which causes malfunction of their cell membrane sodium pump. This results in an influx of sodium and water into cells, and restricted diffusion of intracellular water molecules out of the cells by the cell membranes. The net effect is cell swelling, known as cytotoxic oedema.

Diffusion-weighted imaging (DWI), a specialised form of MRI, makes use of the Brownian motion of water molecules in the brain to generate a signal. Therefore, a high magnitude of molecular diffusion generates a high intensity signal. While classical Brownian motion refers to free movement of molecules, there is restricted movement in biological tissues due to tissue architecture (e.g. cell membranes) and therefore water diffusion is referred to as apparent diffusion. This phenomenon is represented by an image map of the apparent diffusion coefficient (ADC), whereby restricted diffusion generates a low intensity signal.

In the acute ischaemic setting, the restricted diffusion causing cytotoxic oedema results in a low ADC and high DWI signal intensity. This method of diagnostic imaging is very helpful to distinguish acute infarction from old established infarcts.

Intracranial tumours

MRI is more sensitive and specific than CT imaging in detecting and evaluating brain tumours. Intracranial tumours such as meningioma, ependymoma, astrocytoma and metastases are appreciated as isointense or low signal intensity on T1-weighted images and high signal intensity on T2-weighted images, with high signal secondary to the surrounding vasogenic oedema (see Chapter 39). Imaging after injection of gadolinium is a mainstay of imaging intracranial tumours with MRI as most brain tumours cause disruption of the blood–brain barrier and readily take up the contrast agent.

44.1 Lateral XR: normal

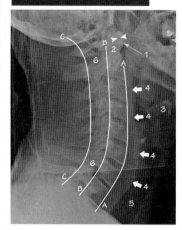

The cervical vertebrae are visible down to T1. The anterior (A), posterior (B) and spinolaminar (C) spinal lines are aligned normally. There is no injury of the bones or prevertebral soft-tissue (4). The atlanto-axial distance is normal (arrowheads)

44.2 Sagittal CT: normal

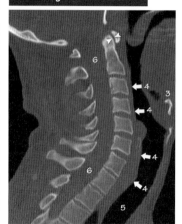

CT appearances of the same patient as in fig 44.1. Normal alignment is shown with no evidence of bone or soft tissue injury. Here the atlanto-axial space (arrowheads) is seen clearly

44.3 AP XR: normal

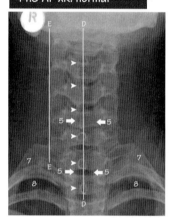

The spinous processes (line D) are normally aligned and equally spaced (arrowheads). The lateral alignment (line E) is also normal on both sides

Key		
1	Atlas (C1)	Lines
2	Odontoid peg of axis (C2)	A Anterior spinal line
3	Hyoid bone	B Posterior spinal line
4	Prevertebral soft tissues	C Spinolaminar line
5	Trachea	D Spinous process line
6	Spinal canal (contains spinal cord)	E Lateral margin line
7	First rib	
8	Lung apex	
9	Teeth	
10	Occipital bone	
11	Spinous process	

44.4 Odontoid peg view XR: normal

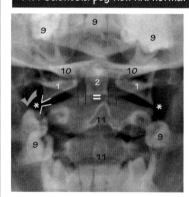

The alignment of the lateral masses of C1 and C2 (*) is normal. The spaces between the peg (2) and the lateral masses of C1 (1) is also equal (red lines). The peg itself is partly obscured by the occipital bone (10)

44.5 Odontoid peg view XR: rotated

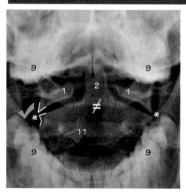

The spaces between the peg (2) and lateral masses of C1 (1) are not equal (red lines). The peg (2) which is an anterior structure does not align with the spinous process (11) which is a posterior structure. The head is rotated with respect to the X-ray beam. Most importantly, however, the lateral masses still show good alignment (*)

Management of cervical spine (C-spine) pathology often requires a combined clinical and radiological approach. In the context of trauma, plain XR imaging may miss significant injury and further imaging with CT and/or MR may be required (see Chapter 45). CT is more sensitive for bony injury and MR for soft tissue injury including ligamentous tears and spinal cord injury. Clinical assessment however should take precedence over imaging, since imaging cannot 'clear' the cervical spine in the context of trauma. If there is clinical suspicion of significant injury without obvious radiological abnormality then assessment by both a senior clinician and a radiologist experienced in neck imaging is required.

Plain XR imaging of the C-spine

The C-spine trauma series includes the following images:
• **Lateral C-spine view** – this view should comprise the entire C-spine (skull base to the superior border of T1). The occipital condyles are seen sitting above the atlas (C1 vertebra) and the mandible lies anteriorly. The C1 vertebra does not have a body but has fused anterior and posterior arches, which are seen framing the dens (odontoid peg) of the axis (C2 vertebra). Below C2 each vertebra consists of a vertebral body, pedicles, superior and inferior articular processes, lamina and a spinous process. The intervertebral disc spaces are normally uniform in height.

The vertebral column has three continuous lines that can be used for assessing alignment:
○ *anterior spinal line* (runs along anterior borders of vertebral bodies)
○ *posterior spinal line* (runs along posterior borders of vertebral bodies)
○ *spinolaminar line* (joins the spinolaminar junctions).
The C-spine can be divided into three individual columns:
○ *anterior column* – anterior longitudinal ligament, and anterior half of vertebral bodies and discs
○ *middle column* – posterior half of vertebral bodies and discs, and posterior longitudinal ligament
○ *posterior column* – posterior elements and multiple associated ligaments.

Disruption of more than one column results in instability, but if only one column is disrupted, the other columns usually provide adequate stability. Columnar disruption may however be present without apparent bony injury on plain XR. Flexion-extension lateral views may help to detect dynamic evidence of ligamentous injury such as 'fanning' of the spinous processes or horizontal movement of one vertebral body on another (spondylolisthesis). The anterior atlanto-axial space should also be checked for widening. This space is normally less than 3 mm in adults and 5 mm in children, and should not change with flexion/extension.

The spinal cord lies in the space between the posterior spinal and spinolaminar lines. The facet joints, which lie immediately behind the posterior spinal line, must be checked to ensure all are visible and align with the opposite side. Each individual vertebral body and posterior element must be assessed for shape, size and cortical breaks and the intervertebral disc spaces should be uniform. The prevertebral soft tissue thickness should measure less than 7 mm above C5 and less than the width of one vertebral body below C5.

Other structures seen on this view include the hyoid bone in the anterior neck and soft tissues, which run along the anterior surface of the vertebral bodies. The soft tissues are seen due to the adjacent contrasting air-filled pharynx, hypopharynx and trachea. The ligaments involved in stabilising the C-spine include the anterior and posterior longitudinal ligaments, which run along the anterior and posterior surfaces of the vertebral bodies respectively; ligamentum flavum, which joins superior and inferior surfaces of adjoining lamina; and interspinous ligaments, which join the spinous processes.
• **Swimmer's view** – this image is usually taken to visualise the lower C-spine more clearly, if obscured on other lateral views. It is taken in a slightly oblique lateral view with one arm up and one down to off set the humeral heads from lying over the cervicothoracic junction. The T1 vertebra normally lies between the clavicle and the first rib on this view.
• **Anteroposterior (AP) C-spine view** – this view is useful in the context of trauma to assess alignment of the spinous processes, which should be aligned and approximately equal distance apart. If the line is discontinuous, unilateral facet joint dislocation should be suspected. If the distance between the processes is widened, vertebral dislocation or ligamentous damage should be suspected.
• **Odontoid peg view** – this view is performed with the patient's mouth open, allowing a direct view of the odontoid peg and atlanto-axial joint. The peg should not be superimposed by teeth or the occiput and the lateral masses of C1 and C2 should be well aligned. The odontoid peg may be considered as the C1 vertebral body, which has fused with C2 and articulates with the anterior arch of C1 in a non-weight-bearing joint. The atlanto-axial joint is strengthened by several ligaments, including the transverse ligament, which passes posteriorly to the peg and holds it in place.
For valid assessment, the head should not be rotated, which is confirmed by inclusion of the lateral borders of C1 and C2, and the equal distance between the peg and the C1 lateral masses. If the head is well centred but there is poor alignment of the C1 lateral masses on C2, this implies a burst fracture of the C1 ring.

CT imaging of the C-spine

CT imaging of the C-spine can be used when there is clinical suspicion of an injury but incomplete plain imaging of the C-spine, or when XR images are normal but high suspicion of injury remains. Alignment, soft tissues and bony structures are carefully assessed. CT is far more sensitive in detecting bony injuries than XR, and may detect soft tissue injuries including prevertebral soft tissue thickening.

MRI of the C-spine

Although C-spine plain XR, flexion-extension views and CT are usually the most useful imaging investigations in the acute setting, if there is clinical evidence of significant soft tissue or neurological injury, MRI should be considered.

45.1 Odontoid peg fracture: peg view

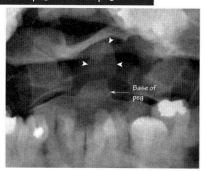

Base of peg

A fracture is seen through the base of the odontoid peg. The tip of the peg is displaced (arrowheads). This is a type 2 odontoid peg fracture

45.2 Jefferson's fracture: peg view

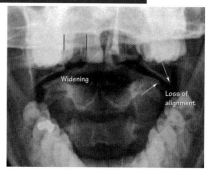

Widening

Loss of alignment

There is widening in the gap between the odontoid peg and the lateral masses of the atlas (red lines). The lateral edges of the atlas/C1 and axis/C2 (arrows) are no longer aligned due to a burst Jefferson-type fracture. Compare with normal alignment (chapter 44)

45.3 C-spine fracture (XR v CT)

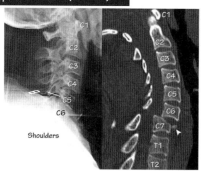

Shoulders

This patient presented with severe lower neck pain and tenderness after a fall downstairs. The lateral XR does not show down to the T1 vertebral body despite several attempts. This is because the shoulders are obscuring the view. A CT of the C-spine (right) revealed a fracture at C7 with malalignment of all three spinal lines

45.4 Rheumatoid arthritis (sagittal T2 MR image)

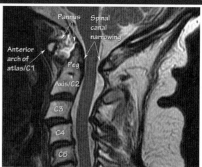

Pannus Spinal canal narrowing

Anterior arch of atlas/C1

Peg

Axis/C2

(Same patient as figs 45.5 and 45.6.) In this patient with chronic rheumatoid arthritis, neck pain and neurological symptoms, there is thick high signal material anterior to the peg. This pannus (synovial thickening) has eroded the peg and destroyed ligaments supporting the atlanto-axial joint, leading to subluxation of this joint (see figs 45.5 and 45.6). This has also caused narrowing of the spinal canal at this level

45.5 Lateral C-spine: extension view

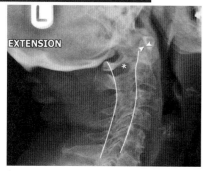

EXTENSION

(Same patient as figs 45.4 and 45.6.) In this position the odontoid peg is shown to be eroded but is closely applied to the anterior arch of the atlas (arrowheads). There is plenty of space in the spinal canal (*) for the spinal cord

45.6 Lateral C-spine: flexion view

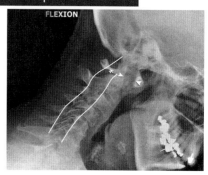

FLEXION

(Same patient as figs 45.4 and 45.5.) On active flexion there is atlanto-axial subluxation (subluxation of the atlas from the axis). The gap between the atlas and the axis (arrowheads) has widened. More significantly the spinal canal (*) is markedly narrowed

Spondylolisthesis

This is abnormal anterior displacement of a vertebral body in relation to the vertebra directly below. It may occur anywhere along the vertebral column, although it is more common in the lumbar region. Spondylolisthesis may be congenital, often presenting in adolescence with lower back pain. Acquired causes include degenerative disease, defects of the pars interarticularis, trauma and pathological spondylolisthesis due to an underlying bone abnormality involving the posterior elements, such as osteoporosis or a malignant lesion. The degree of spondylolisthesis is assessed on the lateral view XR by first measuring the distance between the posterior borders of the displaced vertebral body and the vertebral body directly below, and then expressing this as a percentage of the total displaced vertebral body's AP diameter.

C-spine degenerative disease/osteoarthritis (OA)

The C-spine is a common site for degenerative disease. Patients typically complain of pain in the neck and upper back. If there is impingement of nerve roots as they pass through the exit foramina, there may be pain or other symptoms in the related shoulder, arm or hand.

> ### Classic XR features of C-spine degenerative disease
>
> - Straightened or reversed normal lordosis
> - Intervertebral disc space narrowing
> - Articular surface sclerosis
> - Osteophytes formation (new bone at articular surface edges)
> - Facet joint hypertrophy

Odontoid peg fracture

This is a fracture of the dens (odontoid peg) of the axis (C2 vertebra). The dens articulates with the anterior arch of the atlas (C1 vertebra), which is a non-weight-bearing joint. There are three recognised fracture patterns, which are best seen on an open mouth view XR or CT.

- *Type I* – this is a fracture through the tip of the dens.
- *Type II* – this is a fracture through the base of the dens.
- *Type III* – this is a fracture through the vertebral body of C2.

Hangman's fracture

This injury is caused by forcible hyperextension, often from a blow to the forehead forcing the head into hyperextension. It receives its name from hyperextension of the head during judicial hangings when the body was dropped. The fracture affects both pedicles (pars interarticularis) of the C2 vertebra and is most easily seen on the lateral view or on CT imaging. The fracture does not commonly cause neurological injury, as the spinal canal is actually widened by the separation of the fracture fragments.

Jefferson fracture

This is a compression injury often caused by falls, diving into shallow water, or road traffic accidents. The fracture was first described by the English neurosurgeon Geoffrey Jefferson in 1920. It is a four-part fracture of the anterior and posterior arches of the C1 vertebra. This leads to a widening of the atlas ring and neurological injury is therefore uncommon with this fracture. However, coexisting injuries are common. Fracture variants can include two- or three-part fractures. The fracture is most easily recognised on the peg view, where the lateral masses of C1 (atlas) are laterally displaced with respect to the lateral masses of C2 (axis). There is typically prevertebral soft tissue swelling anterior to C1 on the lateral C-spine view.

Teardrop fracture

This injury is caused by a high-energy flexion force, often seen in head-on vehicle collisions, which results in a fracture of the body of a cervical vertebra. The anterior vertebral body fragment remains attached to the anterior longitudinal ligament and appears as a 'teardrop' on lateral view XR. The remainder of the vertebra is posteriorly distracted and there may be facet joint subluxation with compression of the spinal cord, causing significant neurological impairment (e.g. quadriplegia). This fracture may appear relatively innocent but should be considered highly unstable, with significant risk of associated spinal cord injury.

46.1 Multiple sclerosis: sagittal T2

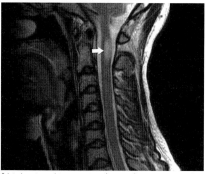

A focus of high signal intensity (arrow) is seen in the spinal cord. Clinically, this patient was suspected to have multiple sclerosis. which was confirmed by further lesions found in the brain

46.2 Cord compression: sagittal T2

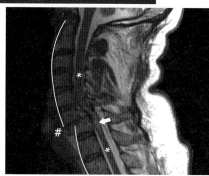

There is discontinuity (#) of the normal alignment due to C-spine fractures at C6 and C7. The spinal canal is markedly narrowed and there is high signal of the cord (arrow) which is a sign of oedema caused by cord injury. Normal cord is seen above and below (*)

46.3 Foraminal narrowing: sagittal and axial T2

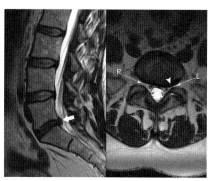

The sagittal image shows a low signal, degenerative and herniated L5/S1 intervertebral disc (short arrow). The axial view shows an intraforaminal protrusion (arrowhead) which is narrowing the left L5 exit foramen (L). Compare with the right (R)

46.4 Sclerotic metastasis: sagittal T2 MR and lateral thoracic XR

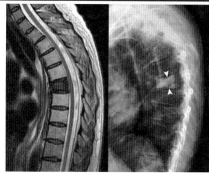

This patient with known breast cancer presented with back pain. There is a single metastasis in a mid-thoracic vertebral body. As the deposit is sclerotic (bony) it demonstrates low signal on all MRI sequences. For comparison the plain XR image shows increased density (arrowheads)

46.5 Cauda equina compression due to discitis: sagittal T2

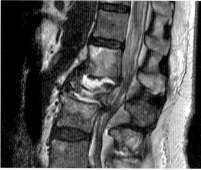

High signal is shown in two intervertebral discs due to infection (discitis) with destruction of the vertebral body between them. There is narrowing of the spinal canal at the level of the cauda equina leading to bilateral perianal and sciatic symptoms in this patient

46.6 Ankylosing spondylitis: sagittal T2 and lateral lumbar XR

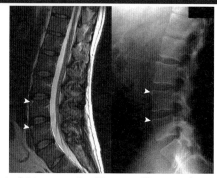

These are the 'shiny corner' or 'Romanus' lesions of early ankylosing spondylitis (arrowheads). The high signal (bright) represents oedema of the underlying marrow whereas the plain XR bright corners represent sclerosis of bone as it heals

MRI has revolutionised spinal imaging due to its excellent demonstration of anatomical structures, high soft tissue definition, and evaluation of pathology. Advantages over CT imaging include accurate assessment of the spinal cord, nerve roots, intervertebral discs and surrounding soft tissues. However, MRI does not allow accurate interpretation of bone cortex abnormalities, which are seen more clearly with XR and CT imaging. Relatively long scan times and the narrower bore of the MR machine compared with CT scanners make MR unsuitable in many acute clinical settings. Claustrophobia and obesity also often prevent the use of MRI. (For other contraindications see Chapter 42.)

MRI of the spine is commonly used for investigating neurological problems such as tumours or multiple sclerosis. Trauma may cause combined neurological and musculoskeletal injury, and MRI is also the primary investigation tool for isolated musculoskeletal problems.

Spinal MRI protocols include sagittal plane T1-weighted and T2-weighted sequences, followed by axial imaging at the level of any abnormality. Short tau inversion recovery (STIR) sequences suppress signal from fat and are sensitive for the presence of abnormal fluid in the bone marrow or intervertebral discs. T1-weighted images, following intravenous injection of gadolinium, may also be performed in order to observe abnormal enhancement of neoplastic or inflammatory tissue anywhere in the spinal column or cord. Image interpretation relies on the different signal intensities of various structures on each sequence (see Chapter 42).

Intervertebral disc herniation

The discs are located between the vertebral bodies and function as shock absorbers. They are composed of a central colloid gel (nucleus pulposus) and a peripheral fibrous capsule (annulus fibrosus). Weakness of the annulus fibrosus allows herniation of the disc substance, which may lead to narrowing of the spinal canal and/or the neural exit foramina. A broad disc herniation (or prolapse) is known as a bulge, whereas a more focal herniation is called a protrusion. An extrusion is a herniation with a narrow base, and a sequestration is an extrusion which has detached from the disc. Herniations may also be classified in terms of their position. They can be central (causing spinal canal narrowing and possible spinal cord or cauda equina compression), paracentral (causing narrowing of the lateral recess of the spinal canal and possible nerve root impingement), intraforaminal (narrowing the exit foramina with potential nerve root impingement) or extraforaminal (which may lead to nerve root impingement outside the spinal canal or exit foramina).

Nerve root compression (radiculopathy)

Herniation of an intervertebral disc is a common cause of back pain and may be accompanied by radicular symptoms (radiculopathy). These are symptoms such as pain, numbness, or weakness caused by impingement of nerve roots as they pass through the neural exit foramina. If there is nerve root impingement in the C-spine, this results in symptoms affecting the respective distribution in the arm. If there is impingement of a nerve root in the lumbar spine (L-spine), sciatic pain results with radiation into the leg. While MRI is highly sensitive for characterising nerve root anatomy, findings on MRI often do not correlate well with the severity of clinical symptoms.

Spinal cord and cauda equina compression

MRI is highly sensitive in assessing narrowing of the spinal canal secondary to disc herniation or other pathology. The degree of spinal canal narrowing can vary from slight indentation of the thecal sac to frank compression of the spinal cord. This may result in neurological signs and symptoms at and below the level of compression.

The spinal cord ends at the conus medullaris (approximately L1–L2). Below this level separate nerve roots descend, which are collectively known as the cauda equina (horse's tail). Spinal canal narrowing at this level may lead to cauda equina syndrome, which clinically manifests as bilateral radicular symptoms in the legs, loss of bladder and/or bowel control, and perianal sensory loss. *This is a neurosurgical emergency.*

Spinal tumours

Primary spinal tumours may originate from any of the local tissue types including bone, cartilage, neural tissue and meningeal tissue. The vertebral column is a common site for bony metastases, such as prostate cancer in men and breast cancer in women.

MRI allows detailed assessment of tumours within the spinal canal itself and may be classified as intradural or extradural (inside or outside the dura). Intradural tumours may be further subdivided into extramedullary (outside cord) or intramedullary (within cord) in origin. Both T1- and T2-weighted images can demonstrate the site, size and margins of the tumour. The tumour composition (solid or cystic), spinal cord oedema and presence of haemorrhage can also be evaluated. As with cerebral tumours, MRI may detect certain characteristics of particular tumour types. However, in reality MRI cannot confidently distinguish between most of the wide range of spinal tumours. Unless there is a known cause of spinal disease, such as a known malignant process with characteristic MRI appearances of metastases, biopsy is often required for accurate diagnosis.

Ankylosing spondylitis

This is a common seronegative (rheumatoid factor negative) arthritis, most frequently affecting men, who present initially with back pain and stiffness. The classic endpoint XR appearance is the so-called 'bamboo spine', caused by ligamentous calcification and vertebral fusion. MRI however plays a role in detecting early signs of ankylosing spondylitis, such as sacroiliitis (inflammation of the sacroiliac joints) or vertebral body 'shiny corners' (the earliest feature of vertebral involvement). As these inflammatory lesions heal, they become sclerotic (bony) and are therefore visible on plain XR imaging of the spine.

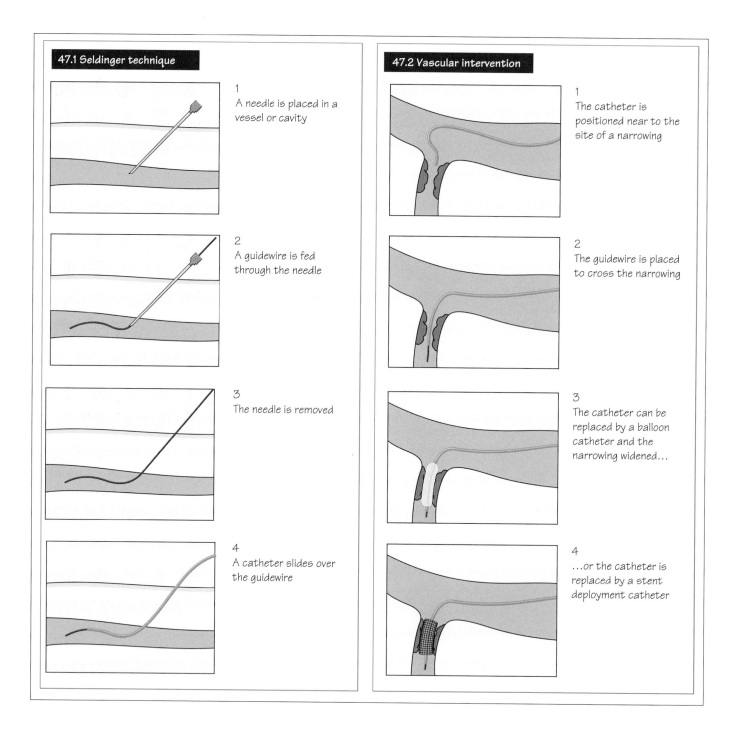

47.1 Seldinger technique

1
A needle is placed in a vessel or cavity

2
A guidewire is fed through the needle

3
The needle is removed

4
A catheter slides over the guidewire

47.2 Vascular intervention

1
The catheter is positioned near to the site of a narrowing

2
The guidewire is placed to cross the narrowing

3
The catheter can be replaced by a balloon catheter and the narrowing widened…

4
…or the catheter is replaced by a stent deployment catheter

Fundamentals of interventional radiology

Interventional radiology (IR) is a rapidly evolving specialty that has impacted on the management of disease in practically all organ systems. It has arisen from the movement towards *minimally invasive therapy* and is the next step on from laparoscopic surgery. While laparoscopic surgery (which uses long and narrow fibreoptic cameras) is called keyhole surgery, IR procedures may be called pinhole surgery. IR procedures use image guidance in the form of ultrasound, fluoroscopy, CT or MR, and often employ the *Seldinger technique*. The usual sequence in an IR procedure therefore begins with the image-guided passage of a needle to a specific target. A guidewire is then passed through the needle and the needle is subsequently removed, leaving the guidewire in situ. Catheters can then be slid over the guidewire to create a direct access port for the procedure or operation. Advances have allowed IR to establish alternatives to traditional operative surgery with equivalence of outcome. A classic example is that of image-guided percutaneous biopsy, which has virtually replaced exploratory laparotomy, the most common surgical procedure of the 1970s. The principal benefits of IR procedures include:

- less anaesthesia
- less pain
- less trauma to the body
- shorter hospital stay
- faster recovery period.

The commonest condition treated by IR is atherosclerosis. Angioplasty and stent placement are therefore one of the most commonly performed IR procedures. Other common procedures are discussed in Chapter 48.

IR is now broadly divided into *vascular* (includes cardiac and neuro-intervention) and *non-vascular intervention*. It should be noted, however, that cardiologists now perform most cardiac interventions.

Interventional radiology checklist

Patients scheduled for an IR procedure should be pre-assessed and worked up in a similar fashion to those undergoing operative surgery. The pre- and post-procedural protocols vary depending on the nature of the procedure performed and local practice.

- **Patient mobility** – the referrer must consider the patient's ability to lie flat and still, and follow instructions.
- **Consent** – patients undergoing any IR procedure must formally consent to the procedure, once they have understood the common risks and benefits of the procedure and been informed of any alternative therapies. Legally, only someone who is qualified to perform the procedure may obtain consent. The spectrum of possible hazards for IR procedures includes: bleeding, infection, embolism, stroke, failure, renal complications, contrast agent reaction, subsequent amputation, surgery and death.
- **Coagulation studies** – all patients undergoing an invasive IR procedure require a recent check of their coagulation status (INR, platelet count) and correction of any coagulopathy before the procedure, to reduce the risk of haemorrhagic complications.
- **Medication** – patients should generally take their regular medication, including their prescribed antihypertensives, as tight blood pressure control is particularly important in angiographic procedures. Anticoagulants, aspirin products, non-steroidal anti-inflammatory drugs and metformin are usually withheld until after the procedure.
- **Sedation and NBM** – many IR procedures are conducted under moderate sedation, e.g. a benzodiazepine. Patients therefore need to be starved at least four hours before some procedures, i.e. nil by mouth (NBM).
- **Hydration** – if patients with impaired renal function require an intravenous iodinated contrast agent for the procedure, they should be hydrated with intravenous fluids before, during, and after the procedure. In some cases the opinion of a renal physician is beneficial prior to a contrast study.
- **Post-procedural checks** – some procedures require the patient to maintain bed rest for several hours after the procedure to minimise the risk of bleeding. The pulses distal to any vascular puncture site should be checked and documented, and any required antibiotics should be prescribed and given.
- **Discharge** – patients must be given adequate analgesia and appropriate post-procedural instructions including wound care advice and instructions for follow-up and emergency. Patients will often also require organised transport and an escort to accompany them home.

48.1 Angioplasty

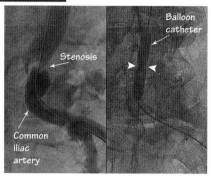

A wire is placed through the stenosis in the common iliac artery. A balloon is inflated to dilate the narrowing (arrowheads). Note: contrast material is black

48.2 IVC filter

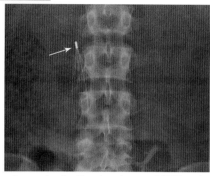

A self-expanding umbrella-like structure or IVC filter (arrow) is placed in the IVC to prevent passage of large emboli to the lungs

48.3 CT-guided biopsy

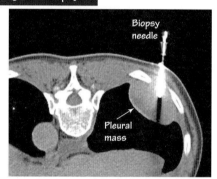

With the patient lying prone a biopsy needle is placed to gain a tissue sample of a large pleural mass

48.4 Colonic stent

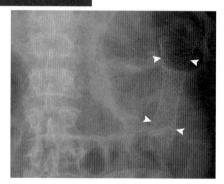

A self-expanding wire-walled stent (arrowheads) is placed via the rectum across an inoperable tumour of the sigmoid colon

48.5 Percutaneous transhepatic cholangiogram (PTC) with biliary stent insertion

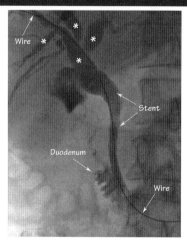

A wire is passed via the liver through a dilated biliary system (*) and into the duodenum. A stent is placed to relieve an obstruction caused by a pancreatic mass

48.6 JJ-ureteric stent

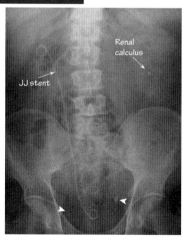

A double pigtail catheter or 'JJ stent' is positioned within the ureter passing from the renal pelvis to the bladder. The patient had recurrent bilateral renal calculi/stones. Multiple phleboliths/venous calcifications (arrowheads) are also seen in the pelvis outside the path of the ureters

Vascular intervention

Vascular interventional radiology has broad applications including the diagnosis and treatment of peripheral vascular disease, aortoiliac disease and aortic aneurysm, renovascular disease, vascular trauma, thromboembolism, pulmonary embolism, tumours, uterine fibroids and portal hypertension. The diagnosis is centred on *percutaneous fluoroscopic angiography* and the therapeutic procedures include:

• **Angioplasty** – this is the balloon dilatation of atherosclerotic vessels, mainly in coronary heart disease and peripheral vascular disease.

• **Stenting** – this is the placement of metal stents to splint open the endovascular lumen.

• **Atherectomy** – this removes atherosclerotic plaques.

• **Aneurysm coil embolisation** – this releases prothrombotic coils into aneurysms (often in the brain) to cause a sealing effect.

• **Endovascular aortic aneurysm repair (EVAR)** – this involves the repair of abdominal aortic aneurysms by deploying stents, which may extended into the iliac vessels depending on the extent of the aneurysm.

• **Embolisation** – this is used to manage bleeding mesenteric vessels or traumatic arterial injuries using a range of materials including coils, beads, gel foam and glue.

• **Uterine artery embolisation** – this is used in the treatment of fibroids (leiomyomas) by selectively blocking their blood supply. This technique offers a less radical treatment option to the surgical alternative of hysterectomy.

• **IVC filter** – an IVC filter fragments large emboli into smaller particles and thereby reduces the risk of massive pulmonary emboli.

• **Thrombectomy** – this removes a thrombus or embolus from an occluded vessel to re-establish blood flow.

• **Transcatheter arterial chemoembolisation (TACE)** – this involves the embolisation of the blood supply and direct administration of chemotherapy to a tumour, e.g. in liver malignancies.

• **Transjugular intrahepatic portosystemic shunt (TIPS)** – this is used in the treatment of portal hypertension where a metal stent is deployed to connect the portal vein to a hepatic vein. This allows portal blood to bypass the liver.

• **Venous port insertion and tunnelled lines** – peripherally inserted central catheters (PICC) and tunnelled lines are inserted under image guidance for the use of long-term antibiotics, chemotherapy and parenteral nutrition.

Non-vascular intervention

Non-vascular interventional radiology has impacted on the management of diseases affecting nearly all organ systems. Common interventions include:

• **Image-guided biopsy** – most parts of the body can be biopsied under image guidance for tissue diagnosis, e.g. lung biopsy.

• **Percutaneous drains** – fluid collections in most parts of the body can be drained under image guidance.

• **Radiofrequency ablation (RFA)** – this is used in the treatment of tumours in the lungs, liver, kidneys, breast and bone. A radiofrequency probe is advanced to the tumour and then radiofrequency waves are applied, which increases the surrounding temperature. This results in targeted and selective tissue destruction of the tumour.

• **Tracheobronchial stenting** – a metal or silicone stent is inserted to splint open an airway narrowed by a malignant obstruction.

• **Oesophageal stenting** – a stent is placed to splint open an oesophageal lumen, narrowed by an obstructing lesion, gastro-oesophageal reflux disease, or post-radiation strictures. It is also used in the treatment of tracheo-oesophageal fistulae.

• **Gastroduodenal stenting** – a metal stent is inserted to splint open the distal stomach or duodenum, narrowed by a malignant obstruction.

• **Colonic stenting** – a metal stent can be sited in the colon to temporarily decompress an acute obstruction from colonic cancer, Crohn's disease, diverticulitis and strictures. Colonic stenting can also be a palliative option in cases of non-resectable colonic cancer.

• **Percutaneous gastrostomy tubes** – these are used in gastric outlet or proximal small bowel obstruction, or for enteral feeding.

• **Percutaneous jejunostomy tubes** – these are used in gastric outlet obstruction or gastric resection.

• **Hepatobiliary intervention** – percutaneous transhepatic cholangiography (PTC) is used to assess biliary obstruction and also allows the relief of an obstruction by biliary duct dilatation, stenting, or the insertion of a drain.

• **Urinary tract intervention** – these therapies include percutaneous nephrostomy to relieve a pyeloureteral obstruction or to drain a renal abscess. Ureteral stenting may be used to relieve an obstruction or contribute to the management of urinary calculi. Percutaneous nephrolithotomy (PCNL) is used to extract and shatter calculi.

• **Musculoskeletal intervention** – these therapies include radiofrequency ablation of bone tumours, nerve root injections with steroid, and vertebroplasty for pain relief in cases of compression fractures and bone tumours (by injecting bone cement to stabilise the fracture).

(49) Principles of nuclear medicine

49.1 Beta decay

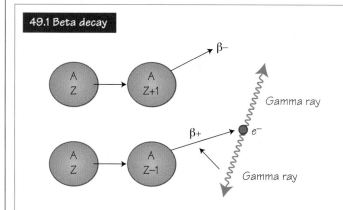

A nucleus that undergoes 'beta minus decay' emits an electron (β-). This forms the basis of many nuclear medicine therapies. A nucleus that undergoes 'beta plus decay' emits a positron (β+) which undergoes annihilation when striking an electron (e-) to emit gamma rays travelling in opposite directions. This forms the basis of PET imaging. Changes in atomic number (Z) and mass number (A) are depicted

49.2 Gamma decay

An excited nucleus that undergoes 'gamma decay' emits a gamma ray and therefore transitions to a more stable state. This forms the basis of most nuclear imaging techniques.

49.3 Gamma camera

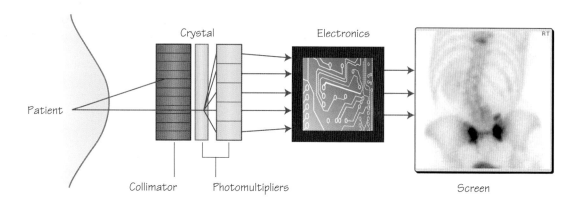

Gamma rays emitted from the patient are collimated to ensure the rays arrive at the crystal in a straight line. The crystal then converts these into photons. The photons are multiplied and converted to electrons which are then converted into an image

Fundamentals of nuclear medicine

Nuclear medicine is a branch of molecular medicine that assesses tissue metabolism and physiology at the cellular and subcellular level to generate images for diagnosis and therapy. A pharmaceutical agent labelled with a radionuclide (radiopharmaceutical) is administered to patients and then gamma cameras detect and measure gamma radiation emitted from the body. The principles of nuclear medicine have many applications in diagnostic imaging.

Physics

Elements are defined by their proton number (atomic number) but their neutron number can vary, giving rise to different isotopes. Atoms with excess or deficient neutrons have unstable nuclei and decay towards a more stable state. These unstable atoms are called radionuclides and can decay in several ways. Beta and gamma decay are used in nuclear medicine.

• *Beta decay* – there are several types of beta decay. 'Beta minus' and 'beta plus' forms of decay are important in nuclear medicine.

Beta minus decay occurs in nuclei with excess neutrons, and involves conversion of a neutron into an electron and proton. The electron is emitted from the nucleus as a beta particle. The mass number stays the same but the atomic number is increased. Iodine-131 (^{131}I) decays to xenon-131 (^{131}X) by beta minus decay and is used in certain nuclear medicine therapies.

Beta plus decay occurs in nuclei with excess protons, and involves conversion of a proton into a neutron, with positron emission (release of a positively charged electron). The positron does not travel far before it interacts with an electron and undergoes 'annihilation', resulting in the emission of two gamma rays, which travel in opposite directions. These gamma rays can travel through body tissues. This forms the basis for positron emission tomography (PET).

• *Gamma decay* – metastable technetium-99 (^{99m}Tc) undergoes gamma decay and is the commonest radionuclide used in diagnostic imaging, e.g. V/Q scan, bone scan, SPECT, MUGA, DMSA, DTPA and MAG3 (see Chapter 50). ^{99m}Tc undergoes the isomeric transition type of gamma decay, where a nucleus in an excited state transitions to a more stable state by emitting a gamma ray.

Most nuclear medicine diagnostic applications use gamma-emitting decay (beta-emitting decay is used in therapeutic applications). Radioactive materials have a half-life that is defined as the time taken for the radioactivity to halve from its original value. The 'effective half-life' is somewhat modified for metabolically active radiopharmaceuticals as it is dependent on the elimination process from the body.

The gamma camera

Radiopharmaceuticals can be injected, ingested or inspired by the patient. Gamma rays are emitted from the body and detected by a crystal that converts them into light. The light signal is then converted into an electrical signal that is displayed on a screen. The brightness of the representative screen pixel is dependent on the number of gamma rays (or counts) detected for a particular volume. The map of the pixels creates an image.

Hazards and precautions

Radiopharmaceuticals can only be prescribed by clinicians who hold an ARSAC licence (see Chapter 6) and must only be handled by licensed technicians. Once patients are administered with a radiopharmaceutical they become radioactive sources until the activity has reached an insignificant level. Certain precautions must therefore be taken during their hospital stay, such as isolation post-injection of a radiopharmaceutical agent, treating all spills (including patient body waste) as radioactive waste, and making patients aware of their potential radioactivity when they leave hospital so they avoid prolonged close contact with children and pregnant women.

50.1 V/Q scan: normal/low probability of pulmonary embolus

L R   R L
LPO Perfusion   ANT Perfusion

L R   R L
LPO Ventilation   ANT Ventilation

The perfusion pattern matches the ventilation pattern. The probability of a significant perfusion defect is therefore low. LPO left posterior oblique, ANT anterior

50.2 V/Q scan: high probability of pulmonary embolus

L R   R L
LPO Perfusion   ANT Perfusion

L R   R L
LPO Ventilation   ANT Ventilation

This patient presented with sudden breathlessness. Ventilation is normal but perfusion is patchy, indicating a high probability of pulmonary embolus. Anticoagulation therapy was initiated

50.3 Bone scan

R   L   L   R
Anterior   Posterior

R Lateral   L Lateral

(Same patient as fig 50.4.) This child presented with left tibial pain, worse at night, and relieved with simple analgesia. These are typical clinical features of an osteoid osteoma. The plain XR showed cortical thickening only. This bone scan shows high uptake of radionuclide material at the site of pain, which indicates an active inflammatory lesion

50.4 CT v PET-CT

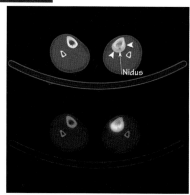

Nidus

(Same patient as fig 50.3.) The CT scan (top) shows the small lucent 'nidus' of an osteoid osteoma (a benign lesion) with surrounding reactive bone formation (arrowheads). The bottom image is a PET/CT scan clearly indicating the location of the active lesion

50.5 Bone scan

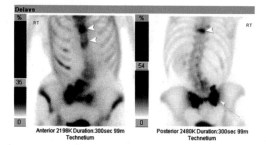

Delays

%   RT
54
35
0
Anterior 2198K Duration:300sec 99m Technetium

%   RT
0
Posterior 2480K Duration:300sec 99m Technetium

This patient with osteoporosis presented with increasing lower back pain. Plain XRs showed vertebral insufficiency fractures which are also seen on these images (arrowheads) but did not reveal the bilateral sacral insufficiency fractures as is evident by uptake in the shape of an H on this scan (Honda sign)

50.6 DMSA: posterior view

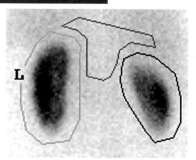

L

This is a DMSA study in a patient with renal artery stenosis. It was performed to determine comparative functional uptake of radionuclide contrast material. In this case the right kidney showed a relative uptake of 42%

Ventilation/Perfusion (V/Q) scanning

V/Q scanning is used to assess the flow of air and blood in the lungs. The ventilation phase involves the patient inspiring xenon or technetium-99m labelled diethylenetriamine pentaacetic acid (^{99m}Tc DTPA) and the perfusion phase involves the injection of technetium-99m labelled macroaggregated albumin (^{99m}Tc MAA). The image series includes anterior, posterior and two posterior oblique projections for both ventilation and perfusion phases. V/Q scans are most commonly used to detect a pulmonary embolus, although in many centres CTPA is now preferentially performed (see Chapter 34). This is partly because underlying or concurrent lung disease reduces the sensitivity and specificity of V/Q scanning. A CXR is performed prior to V/Q scanning to exclude gross lung disease. If the CXR is not normal, a CTPA may be performed after discussion with the radiologist and only if the patient's renal function is adequate. A high probability of pulmonary embolus is interpreted from a V/Q scan that demonstrates a perfusion defect without a corresponding ventilation defect.

Bone scan

Bone scans can detect areas of metabolically abnormal bone. The patient is injected with technetium-99m labelled methylene diphosphonate (^{99m}Tc MDP) and gamma camera imaging is usually performed three to four hours later. There is often normal physiological uptake of radionuclide by the kidneys, breast, bowel and thyroid. However, focal hotspots (high uptake) in bone may be due to primary cancer, metastasis, arthropathy, trauma, osteomyelitis and avascular necrosis. Focal coldspots (low uptake) are often due to restriction of local blood supply (such as sickle cell crisis and post-traumatic avascular necrosis) or a destructive process leading to bone replacement (such as metastasis primarily from the kidney, lung, breast and multiple myeloma).

Positron emission tomography (PET)

PET is based on beta plus decay of an injected radionuclide (see Chapter 49), most commonly ^{18}F fluorodeoxyglucose (FDG), which is a glucose analogue. The uptake of FDG is proportional to local glucose metabolism and gamma cameras surround the patient to detect the emitted rays. For each annihilation event, two gamma rays are emitted, travelling in opposite directions. Each of these rays is detected within a short time window of each other by a camera. By measuring the time difference between the detection of each ray by the two opposing cameras, the position of the original annihilation event can be mapped. This is then used to construct an image.

One of the most rapidly developing areas of radiology is PET/CT where PET imaging is performed in conjunction with CT imaging to combine functional and anatomical data. The commonest application is in the detection and evaluation of primary tumours and metastases. Most cancers have a high metabolism and consequently have increased uptake of FDG compared to normal tissue. Primary and metastatic cancers therefore stand out as hotspots on PET and PET/CT.

Single photon emission computed tomography (SPECT)

SPECT resembles the technique of conventional CT. It involves a rotating gamma camera, which detects counts at multiple projections and at set angles of travel. The two-dimensional information is then resolved into a three-dimensional data set. Typical applications include myocardial perfusion scanning to evaluate myocardial ischaemia, and functional brain imaging. Commonly used radiopharmceuticals include thallium-201 and technetium-99m labelled agents.

Gated cardiac blood-pool imaging

This nuclear medicine technique is also known as multigated acquisition (MUGA) imaging and involves labelling the patient's red blood cells with technetium-99m, which then circulate within the body's blood pool. Gamma camera images of the heart are 'gated' (acquired in synchrony with the cardiac cycle), so that the detected gamma radiation can be mapped to each stage of the cycle. This technique is primarily used to evaluate cardiac ventricular function.

Renal imaging

Nuclear medicine imaging of the kidneys is commonly used to evaluate renal function and anatomy. Common techniques include:
- **Static renal scan (DMSA scan):** This nuclear medicine technique is used to determine renal size, shape and position. It therefore provides information regarding renal structure in suspected horseshoe, solitary, or ectopic kidneys. It is also valuable in assessing renal parenchymal abnormalities including acute pyelonephritis and scarring post infection (particularly in children with proven urinary tract infections). The patient is injected with technetium-99m labelled dimercaptosuccinic acid (^{99m}Tc DMSA), which binds to functioning proximal tubular cells, and gamma camera imaging is performed several hours later.
- **Dynamic renal scans:** These techniques are used to evaluate specific areas of renal function.
  - DTPA scanning – this nuclear medicine technique is used to assess renal glomerular filtration, renal tract obstruction and vesicoureteric reflux. Technetium-99m labelled diethylenetriamine pentaacetic acid (^{99m}Tc DTPA) is injected and gamma camera images are taken over the next 30 minutes.
  - MAG3 scanning – this nuclear medicine technique is used to assess the function of the renal tubules, collecting ducts and renal blood flow. It has many applications including detecting renal artery stenosis in kidney donors pre-transplantation. The technique is based on tracking the passage of intravenously administered technetium-99m labelled mercaptoacetyltriglycine (^{99m}Tc MAG3) through the kidney.

Classic nuclear medicine applications

V/Q scan	Pulmonary embolus
Bone scan	Primary bone cancer, metastatic bone cancer, arthropathy, trauma, osteomyelitis and avascular necrosis
PET	Primary cancer and metastasis
SPECT	Myocardial perfusion imaging, functional brain imaging, cancer
MUGA	Cardiac ventricular function
DMSA	Congenital renal abnormalities, acute pyelonephritis, renal scarring
MAG3	Renal blood flow, renal tubular and ductal function, drainage

Radiology OSCE, case studies and questions

OSCE principles

OSCEs (objective structured clinical examinations) are the source of much anxiety for medical students, but in reality are a relatively straightforward part of medical finals. Many students believe they have to show great expertise during the OSCE, but often the scenarios set are designed to ensure that you pass if you are safe to practise, and fail only if you are dangerous or impolite.

Radiology is now examined as a core subject by many medical schools, and the principles that apply to many OSCE scenarios also apply to radiology.

Many of the chapters in this book have been designed to give you an approach to interpreting a wide range of imaging studies. These approaches can be used in clinical practice but, perhaps equally importantly, having an approach is essential for scoring highly in the OSCE setting. You certainly do not have to learn all these approaches, and in fact there are very few scenarios that are likely to come up in a finals OSCE. The scenario must test core skills. It would therefore be unfair to expect you to interpret complex CT, MRI or US examinations. Examiners set scenarios that allow you not only to pass, but also to shine if you are a good candidate, and fail if you fall below a minimum required standard. There are therefore only a limited number of clinical scenarios which are fair to include. You should never be expected to be a radiological expert, and often the questions you are given within the OSCE will relate more to the clinical setting in which the image has been taken. You are likely to be asked about other investigations that may be helpful and how management is changed by the information provided by the radiological test.

Typical radiology OSCE scenarios

Chest	Pneumothorax (Chapter 13)
	Pleural effusion (Chapter 12)
	Lung cancer (Chapter 14)
Abdomen	Bowel obstruction (Chapter 17)
	Bowel perforation (Chapter 17)

For each station you will be given a minute or two to consider a clinical scenario relating to the images you will be asked to interpret and comment on. You should keep this information at the forefront of your mind, and often you will have the answer, or at least a very good idea of what to expect, before you even set eyes on an image. Typically you will be asked to present an X-ray, describing what you see as you go, and to summarise your findings, suggesting further investigations or management. Poor candidates need prompting at every stage, and find it difficult to link the imaging to the clinical scenario. Good candidates can score all the points without ever being asked a question as they have continued to talk and already answered them appropriately. Most candidates fall somewhere in the middle, sometimes needing prompting and sometimes taking the initiative.

It is generally true that examiners are on your side and there is nothing they dislike more than failing a candidate. You should therefore always follow prompts when they are given. For example, if you are asked 'Is there a tension pneumothorax?', you had better be sure there isn't one before you say 'No'. This is the quickest way to fail the OSCE. Also, whatever you do *never* argue with the examiner, and *always* thank him/her at the end. Although you are unlikely to have patient contact in the radiology station, the only other way of quickly failing an OSCE station is to harm a patient or be discourteous. You must also therefore *always* thank any patient you come into contact with, and respect their dignity by replacing any clothing you have removed. Don't forget that in the radiology OSCE you have equal, if not more, potential to harm the patient if you get it wrong. It is a good principle to treat a radiographic image as a patient, not merely as a picture. Don't forget, a picture of bowel perforation represents a real event happening to a real patient.

You may find it useful to practise the following examples in a group, with one person acting as examiner, one as examinee and others as observers. Use the examiner's checklist here and give marks for your answers to each question, suggesting how these answers could be improved.

Examiner's checklist

ID examination (e.g. PA chest radiograph)
ID patient (name)
State date X-ray taken
Comment on technical quality
Describe what you see as you are going
At the end summarise your findings in one sentence
Suggest diagnosis
Suggest immediate clinical management

CXR	Artefacts or foreign bodies
	Describe any obvious abnormality
	Trachea (central?)
	Lung zones (symmetry?)
	Mediastinum (e.g. aortic knuckle)
	Heart size
	Costophrenic angles (sharp?)
	Hemidiaphragms (well-defined?)
	Bones and soft tissues
AXR	Describe any obvious abnormality
	Bowel gas pattern (dilatation?)
	Abnormal calcification (e.g. stones)
	Bones and soft tissues
IVU	Control image (stones?)
	Delay of contrast uptake into kidneys
	Delay of excretion into ureters
	Column of contrast post micturition

Case 1

(allow 1 minute to read this information)

You are an F1 doctor passing through the busy Emergency Department on your first medical on-call. You are asked to look at a chest X-ray by a radiographer, who can't find another doctor. You know nothing about the patient and are expected on the ward to take some blood. As the radiographer seems worried and tells you the patient seems very short of breath, you take a look at the X-ray.

Please present the X-ray and summarise your findings.

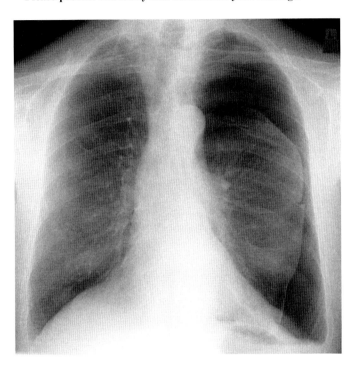

Case 1 Presentation and summary of findings
Include points from examiner's checklist (see p. 110).
- Large left-sided pneumothorax
- Evidence of tension (see answer to question 6)
- No visible rib fractures
- No evidence of underlying lung disease

Case 1 Additional OSCE questions
1 *What is the immediate management for this patient?*
2 *What types of pneumothorax do you know?*
3 *How is a large pneumothorax defined?*
4 *Which medical conditions predispose to pneumothorax?*
5 *What are the clinical signs of a tension pneumothorax?*
6 *Is this a tension pneumothorax?*
Honours question
7 *Where would you find current guidelines for the management of a pneumothorax?*

Case 2

(allow 1 minute to read this information)

You see a patient in the Outpatient Department. Previous medical history includes a right hemicolectomy for a colon cancer one year ago. The patient has come in for a routine check, but complains of gradually increasing shortness of breath. On examination you note that the patient is tachypnoeic and tachycardic at rest with poor air entry at the lung bases. While you send the patient off for a chest X-ray you notice that recent blood tests show abnormal liver function tests.

Please present the X-ray and summarise your findings.

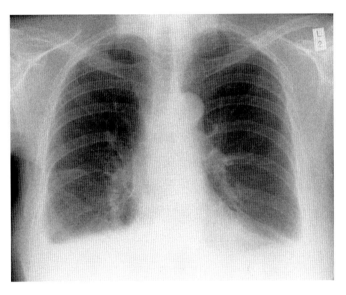

Case 2 Presentation and summary of findings
Include points from examiner's checklist (see p. 110).
- Bilateral pleural effusions with 'meniscus sign' with increased fluid in the horizontal fissure
- Normal heart size
- Normal underlying lung parenchyma and lung volume

Case 2 Additional OSCE questions
1 *What clinical signs would you expect in this patient?*
2 *What is the likely cause of the pleural effusions in this patient with abnormal liver function tests?*
3 *What is the difference between a transudate and an exudate?*
4 *What other causes of pleural effusions do you know?*
5 *How would you manage this patient?*
6 *Which other imaging investigations may be helpful?*
Honours question
7 *What are the CXR features of pulmonary disease in rheumatoid arthritis?*

Case 3

(allow 1 minute to read this information)

You are working at night on your first surgical on call. You are asked by your registrar to assess a woman who is unwell. You are not sure why you have been asked to see her and when you get there she is difficult to assess because she is confused and unaccompanied. A nurse gives you the Emergency Department notes which you can't read, but you can see that the patient has never had an operation and that a request has gone to the X-ray department.

Please present the X-ray and summarise your findings.

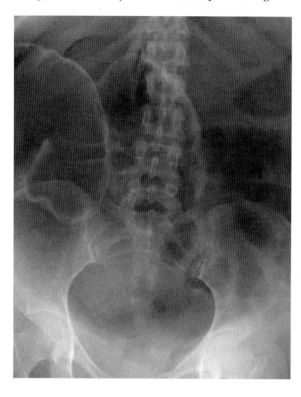

Case 3 Presentation and summary of findings

Include points from examiner's checklist (see p. 110).

- Dilated loops of small and large bowel
- Empty rectum
- Both sides of the bowel wall are visible
- Free edge of gas outlining the liver
- There is large bowel obstruction complicated by perforation

Case 3 Additional OSCE questions

1 *What investigation would you request next and what would you expect to see?*
2 *What clinical symptoms and signs would you expect?*
3 *What are the causes of bowel obstruction?*
4 *What is the immediate management for this patient?*
5 *Which other imaging investigations would be most helpful?*

Honours question

6 *What precautions should be taken before giving IV contrast?*

Please present the X-ray and summarise your findings.

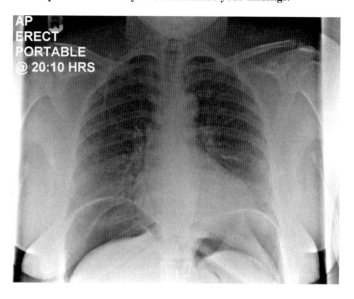

Case 3 (continued) Presentation and summary of findings

Include points from examiner's checklist (see p. 110).

- Comment specifically on the radiograph being 'erect'
- Air under diaphragm forming crescents
- Pneumoperitoneum in keeping with perforation
- Normal lungs
- You will be marked down if you state that the heart is big (it is an AP view and so the heart size is exaggerated)

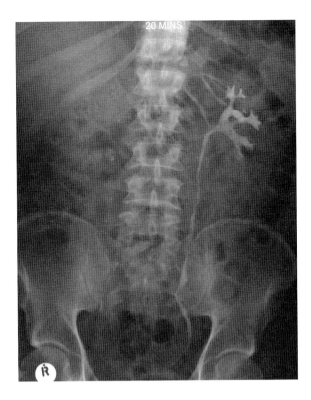

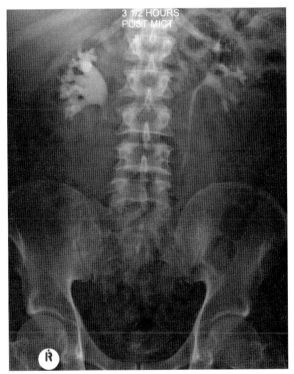

Case 4

(allow 1 minute to read this information)

You are asked to assess a middle-aged man with a family history of abdominal pain. When you meet him he is in severe pain and cannot keep still. An imaging investigation is under way.

Please present the X-rays and summarise your findings.

Case 4 Presentation and summary of findings

Include points from examiner's checklist (see p. 110).

- 20 minute and 3.5 hour IVU images
- Ask for control image (adds no information in this case)
- Normal left pelvicalyceal system (PCS) and ureter
- No contrast seen in right PCS or ureter at 20 minutes indicating ureteric obstruction
- Possible stone adjacent to right L3 transverse process seen on 20-minute image
- Dilated (clubbed) PCS above level of L3 stone on the 3.5 hour image indicating obstruction

Case 4 Additional OSCE questions

1 *Prior to imaging, which bedside tests may be helpful?*
2 *What is the (a) initial, (b) longer-term and (c) preventive management of a patient with renal colic?*
3 *What other imaging tests can be used in this situation?*
4 *What percentage of renal stones are radio-opaque?*

Honours question

5 *Which stones are radiolucent?*

Answers

Case 1

1 *What is the immediate management for this patient?*
- Locate the patient immediately
- Assess – **a**irways, **b**reathing and **c**irculation
- Call for immediate nursing and senior medical help
- Give oxygen
- Aspirate with a cannula placed in the second anterior intercostal space in the mid-clavicular line on the left
- Repeat if fails
- Gain IV access
- Gain history from notes and patient
- Organise chest drain/admission/discussion with respiratory physicians

2 *What types of pneumothorax do you know?*
- Small/Large (see answer 3)
- Open (air sucked in through hole in chest wall)
- Tension (see answer 6)
- Hydropneumothorax/haemopneumothorax *(see chapter 13)*
- Primary/secondary (lung disease)
- Traumatic (due to rib fractures or sharp injury)

3 *How is a large pneumothorax defined?*
- >2 cm from lung edge to chest wall

4 *What factors predispose to pneumothorax?*
- Tall/young/male/smoker (spontaneous)
- Underlying lung disease (fibrosis, pneumonias including PCP, asthma, and COPD)
- Ventilated patients
- Chest wall injury

5 *What are the clinical signs of a tension pneumothorax?*
- Tachypnoea/cyanosis/hypotension/distended neck veins
- Deviated trachea away from affected side
- Poor chest expansion on affected side
- Hyper-resonance to percussion on affected side
- Reduced breath sounds on affected side

6 *Is this a tension pneumothorax?*
- Yes. The trachea and heart appear pushed to the right. This is exaggerated by patient rotation, making accurate assessment of mediastinal deviation difficult. There is nevertheless evidence of tension, indicated by depression of the left hemidiaphragm. A good student will point this out. An average student will comment that the pneumothorax is large (>2 cm) and will need treatment anyway. The student who wants to fail will suggest there is no need to reassess the patient and insists on repeating the X-ray.

7 *Where would you find guidelines for management of a pneumothorax?*
- The British Thoracic Society website http://www.brit-thoracic.org.uk

Case 2

1 *What clinical signs may you find in this patient?*
- Tachypnoea/tachycardia
- 'Stony' dullness to percussion bibasally
- Reduced/absent breath sounds at the lung bases
- Reduced vocal resonance and tactile vocal fremitus
- Bronchial breathing at the top of the effusions
- Normal breath sounds above the effusions
- Hepatomegaly and/or stigmata of liver disease
- General signs of malignancy such as cachexia
- Peripheral oedema and ascites

2 *What is the likely cause of the pleural effusions in this patient with abnormal liver function tests?*
- Low protein (albumin) due to liver metastases

3 *What is the difference between a transudate and an exudate?*
- Transudate = protein concentration of <30 g/L
- Exudate = protein concentration of >30 g/L

4 *What other causes of pleural effusions do you know?*
- Transudate
  Increased venous pressure
  Heart failure/pericardial disease
  Fluid overload
  Decreased oncotic pressure
  Liver failure
  Nephrotic syndrome
  Malnutrition
- Exudate
  Infection (empyema if contains pus)
  Malignancy
  Connective tissue disease
  Rheumatoid arthritis
  Systemic lupus erythematosus
- Other
  Haemothorax
  Chylothorax

5 *How would you manage this patient?*
- Assess ABC and obtain senior advice
- Give oxygen and transfuse if required
- Aspiration or drainage if the patient is symptomatic
- Send sample for biochemistry, cytology (microbiology and immunology are not required in this case but may be necessary if infection or connective tissue disease suspected)
- Consider further imaging (see question 6)
- Treat underlying cause
- If metastasis is confirmed inform patient and oncology

6 *Which other imaging investigations may be helpful?*
- CXR after aspiration/insertion of chest drain
- US of the abdomen to confirm liver metastases/ascites
- Chest US to confirm pleural effusions and guide aspiration drainage
- CT chest, abdomen and pelvis for restaging of cancer

7 *What are the CXR features of pulmonary disease in rheumatoid arthritis?*
- Pleural effusions
- Fibrosis
- Pulmonary nodules
- Cardiomegaly (pericarditis with pericardial effusion)
- Enlarged pulmonary arteries (pulmonary hypertension)
- Shoulder disease (erosions or secondary osteoarthritis)

Case 3

1 *What investigation would you request next and what would you expect to see?*
- An 'erect' chest X-ray
- Free intra-abdominal gas collecting under the diaphragm

2 *What symptoms and signs would you expect?*
- Symptoms:
  Vomiting
  Severe abdominal pain
  Absolute constipation
- Signs:
  Tachycardia, shallow breathing
  Abdominal guarding, tenderness
  Tympanic percussion note on abdomen
  'Tinkling' or absent bowel sounds

3 *What are the causes of bowel obstruction?*
- Hernia
- Adhesions
- Tumours (cause in this case)
- Volvulus
- Intussusception
- Strictures (diverticular disease or IBD)
- Gallstone ileus
- Foreign body

4 *What is the immediate management for this patient?*
- IV fluid (drip) and nasogastric tube (suck)
- Analgesia
- Plan for surgery

5 *Which other imaging investigations would be most helpful?*
- A gastrografin enema (insertion of gastografin contrast via a rectal catheter to assess level of obstruction)
- CT of the abdomen and pelvis (with IV contrast enhancement) is the investigation of choice to assess the level of obstruction and the cause

6 *What precautions should be taken before giving IV contrast? (see chapter 6)*
- Allergy history
- Diabetic history (increased risk of nephrotoxicity and if on metformin this will need to be stopped and renal function checked before restarting)
- Assess renal function and balance risk against potential gain of performing the scan
- IV hydration in sick patients

Case 4

1 *Prior to imaging which bedside tests may be helpful?*
- Renal function prior to giving intravenous contrast
- Urine dipstick to check for haematuria

2 *What is the (a) initial, (b) longer-term and (c) preventive management of a patient with renal colic?*
- (a) Initial
  - Analgesia (opiates often required)
  - Fluids
  - Filter urine to catch passing stones for assessment
  - Allow stone to pass if less than 5 mm
  - Inform urologist
- (b) Longer term
  - Nephrostomy
  - Endoscopic removal
  - Percutaneous surgery
  - Extracorporeal shockwave lithotripsy (use of ultrasound to fragment stones – used for upper tract stones only)
- (c) Prevention
  - Increase fluid intake
  - Avoid dehydration
  - Control metabolic imbalance if present

3 *What other imaging tests can be used in this situation?*
- Ultrasound can assess for pelvi-calyceal dilatation but is limited in determining the level of obstruction
- CT KUB is the investigation of choice in renal colic patients and can determine causes other than renal stones

4 *What percentage of renal stones are radio-opaque?*
- 90% (calcium-containing stones)

5 *Which stones are radiolucent?*
- Cysteine, uric acid, xanthine, matrix

Index

Note: page numbers in *italics* refer to figures and boxes